PHYSIOLOGY - LABORATORY AND CLINICAL RESEARCH

RESTLESS LEGS SYNDROME AND PERIODIC LEG MOVEMENTS

NEUROPLASTICITY INSIGHTS AND PHYSIOTHERAPEUTIC APPROACH

A GUIDE FOR PHYSIOTHERAPISTS

PHYSIOLOGY – LABORATORY AND CLINICAL RESEARCH

PHYSIOLOGY - LABORATORY AND CLINICAL RESEARCH

RESTLESS LEGS SYNDROME AND PERIODIC LEG MOVEMENTS

NEUROPLASTICITY INSIGHTS AND PHYSIOTHERAPEUTIC APPROACH

A GUIDE FOR PHYSIOTHERAPISTS

SUSANA TELLES

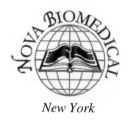

New York

Library of Congress Cataloging-in-Publication Data

ISBN: 978-1-63117-926-6

Library of Congress Control Number: 2014945912

Published by Nova Science Publishers, Inc. † *New York*

Contents

Preface

My story in the field of Sleep began in the first year of a Physiotherapy Course in Universidade de São Paulo, more specifically in neuroanatomical studies when I first learned about reticular formation, connected both to sleep and movements. I stored that amazing information until the end of my *latu sensu* in Neurological Disorders, when I read a revision linking motor learning and sleep. Almost at the same time, I took Bobath Baby course. It was during one of the introductory classes that the teacher asked if there was anyone interested in sleep...and I was the only one raising a hand.

From that time on, Dr. Rosana Alves from the Bobath course became my instructor during my master's degree and introduced me to the field of Sleep and Periodic Leg Movements in subjects with spinal cord injury. From the moment I started to go to Sleep Congresses in Brazil, I didn´t feel so alone, although there were only a few physiotherapists working in the field.

Nowadays I am the president of the Physiotherapy Department in the Brazilian Sleep Association. I have been working to gather colleagues throughout this continental country to bring more physiotherapists to the Sleep field, and to warn our colleagues and professors how important Sleep is in Physiotherapy.

This book is a collection of possible interventions for patients afflicted by Restless Legs Syndrome and Periodic Leg Movements Disorder that physiotherapists can apply. For that the physiotherapist must know the basic physiology of sleep, the physiopathology of those disorders, the proper exam and diagnosis, and the medicines that are used to treat this disorder.

Finally, my hope is that the knowledge in this book will spread and I, hopefully in twenty-five years from now, can read this preface and be glad that the physiotherapists did enter into the Sleep field, in my country and others, so that patients with Restless Legs Syndrome and Periodic Leg Movements Disorder can be treated by physiotherapists accordingly.

Dr. Susana Telles
R. Capote Valente, n.302 – Jardim Paulista São Paulo, SP
CEP: 05409-000
Tel: 02111 991957006
E-mail: telles.susana@gmail.com

Acknowledgments

I thank my family for their support; especially my parents who stimulated my learning and interaction in the English language.

I thank Dr. Rosana Alves and Professor Gerson Chadi for guiding my steps trough the mysteries of neuroplasticity and sleep. I thank all of the students involved in those studies in Universidade de São Paulo at that time in LIM45. I thank also Professor Rogério Silva and many others involved in teaching me the basics of Sleep Physiology. I thank the Brazilian Sleep Association for supporting the Physiotherapists in the Sleep field. I thank Professor Clarice Tanaka and Professor Amélia Pasqual Marques for supporting the Sleep field in Physiotherapy. I thank my colleagues from the Physiotherapy department in the Brazilian Sleep Association for their support.

I thank, *in memoriam*, three great professors whom I had the honor to meet: Dr. Flávio Aloe, Dr. Sonia Gusman and Dr. Odete de Fátima Durigon. I humbly try to follow in your footsteps. Your teaching has touched me deeply, marked my development and made me go on researching Restless Legs Syndrome, Periodic Leg Movements and all sleep disorders.

Chapter 1

Sleep Physiology Overview

Abstract

In this chapter the reader will read an overview of sleep physiology. 1. The reader will be introduced to important concepts such as regular sleep architecture: concept, daily application, brief introduction to circadian disturbances. 2. Sleep stages: Sleep deprivation: expected amount of sleep at each age, brief introduction to sleep deprivation. 3. The concept of circadian rhythms and circadian disorders including Restless Legs Syndrome. Also, the reader will learn the amount of sleep we should all have and there will be a brief discussion about sleep deprivation and its consequences to health since this an important issue in Restless Legs Syndrome patients. Finally, there will be a brief introduction about physiotherapists´ daily practice in Brazil in the Sleep field.

Introduction to Sleep and Physiotherapy

a. Regular Sleep: Architecture and Sleep Stages

Sleep Science is a young part of Science in the world, having been considered scientific research material only in the last 50 years. Those researches approached animals and humankind because all species have this consciousness alteration to rest in a 24-hour period. The electroencephalogram was then essential to stand for two main concepts: there is neural activity during sleep and it is standardized inside the species and in percentage of time [1].

In humankind, there are NREM (non-rapid eye movements) formed by stages 1, 2 and 3 and the REM (rapid eye movements) sleep. Stage 1 is the transition from wake to sleep, characterized by 12 Hz waves and slow eye movements. Stage 2 is characterized by k complex (low potential followed by a high potential) and sleep spindles (conjunction of higher frequency waves). Stage 3 is formed by low frequency and higher amplitude waves, being present mainly during the first half of the night. REM sleep is characterized by desynchronized low frequency action potentials, and muscular atonia except for the eye muscles. Nowadays, magnetic resonance techniques show which part of the brain is active during each sleep stage [2].

The hypnogram is a graphic obtained during sleep study. This graphic shows in the y axis the types of sleep and in the x axis the time of the night.

As a fetus and into early childhood, there is a large proportion of REM sleep and 10 or 12 hours of sleep is considered normal. After two years of age, stage 2 increases in percentage, while sleep duration decreases until adulthood. In older age, sleep becomes more fragmented during the 24-hour period.

b. Circadian Rhythms: Concept, Daily Application, Brief Introduction to Circadian Disturbances

Circadian rhythms are the physiological occurrence of specific behaviors repeated in the same moment during the daylight cycles and 24-hour period. Sleep is entrained in a certain period so all other behaviors related to physical activity are entrained in the opposite period. In humans this includes hormone liberation, immunological activity, digestive system activity, cardiac, respiratory, and muscular and neurological oscillations, all due according to this body schedule.

Circadian disorders can occur due to genetic predisposition, work shift, other health disorders or bad sleep habits. These include early phase disorder, late phase disorder, and free course disorder. In the early phase, the person feels sleepy around 8:00 p.m. and wakes up around 4:00 a.m. In the late phase disorder, the person goes to bed around 2:00 a.m. and wakes up around 10:00 a.m.

Shift work is related to several increased risks of diseases such as breast cancer [3]. It also disturbs the social interactions of the individual and it causes other sleep disorders such as insomnia. There are many accidents linked to the decreased attention caused by night shifts.

Restless Legs Syndrome has a strong circadian character [4]. The symptoms start in the evening, and continue during the first half of the night. This is one of the features that marks and defines this disorder. There are other health disorders that are connected to a marked circadian symptomatology such as rheumatoid arthritis, which is characterized by pain in the morning.

c. Sleep Duration: Sleep Deprivation: Expected Amount of Sleep at Each Age; Brief Introduction to Sleep Deprivation

Humankind has sleep entrained in the dark period, while activity and daylight come together [5]. Babies can sleep 12 hours a day, while young adults usually sleep about 7 hours a day. In older ages, our sleep tends to be fragmented during the day. REM sleep occupies the majority sleeping period when we are babies, and after two years of age, delta waves take their place until we become adults, when stages 1 and 2 are also present.

There is no rule concerning how many hours humans should sleep. What is known so far is that some people are genetically prone to sleep four hours a night and others need 10 hours a night as adults.

Sleep deprivation is a social/biological phenomenon that can occur sporadically or in chronic fashion. It is a characteristic of modern society which works 24 hours a day. The alarming tendency of not getting enough sleep is seen in all ages and it carries vicious consequences such as diurnal somnolence, lack of attention, and diminished concentration. In the long run, patients tend to have more risk of hypertension [6] or cancer. Health professionals should alert all patients to the risks inherent in chronic sleep deprivation and should advise and orient good sleep habits.

Sleep deprivation is related to Restless Legs Syndrome because of its circadian marked rhythm. Actually, this is considered a functional consequence, as the person afflicted with those symptoms late at night is doomed to be chronically sleep deprived.

d. Sleep Disorders and Physiotherapy: Brief Introduction to Physiotherapy Daily Practice in Sleep Disorders

This section regards physiotherapy practice in Brazil only. Each country has its own sleep therapists in the field.

In Brazil physiotherapists can work in sleep laboratories as sleep technologists to perform basal polysomnography and titration. They can work the night shift monitoring the patients directly or they can work by reading polysomnography tests. This work is followed by a sleep doctor's revision.

The physiotherapist also works in CPAP adaptation, selling devices and masks for sleep apnea patients.

Sleep science is not yet inserted into our undergraduate courses. It could be applied in our daily practice from the Intensive Therapy Unit and daily ambulatory care in the usual physiotherapy patients. Sleep health is very important for better results in dealing with stroke and cardiac patients, or musculoskeletal pain afflicted subjects.

There is not yet a specific post-graduate course in the area, so many physiotherapists who work in the field were trained inside companies; others completed a master's degree or PhD in the area, learning Sleep Science at university. Scientific works usually focus on sleep apnea syndrome and CPAP adherence or sleep quality in physiotherapy patients, used as a tool to show the efficacy of physiotherapy treatment. Actigraphy, an accelerometer that registers physical activity, is also a very common tool in physiotherapy scientific works.

It is a new area and there are few professionals working in the field. It requires urgent expansion because the Brazilian population suffers from many sleep disorders. Physiotherapists and other health professionals are not familiar with Restless Legs Syndrome in Brazil, so patients are probably underdiagnosed and not treated at all.

References

[1]   Dement WC. History of Sleep Physiology and Medicine. In: Kryger MH, Roth T, Dement WC, editors. *Principles and Practice of Sleep Medicine.* 1. 5th ed. Canada: Elsevier; 2011. p. 6-9.

[2]   Maquet P. Functional neuroimaging of normal human sleep by positron emission tomography. *Journal of sleep research.* 2000;9(3):207-31.

[3]   Hansen J, Stevens RG. Case-control study of shift-work and breast cancer risk in Danish nurses: impact of shift systems. *European journal of cancer* (Oxford, England: 1990). 2012;48(11):1722-9.

[4]   Hening WA, Walters AS, Wagner M, Rosen R, Chen V, Kim S, et al. Circadian rhythm of motor restlessness and sensory symptoms in the idiopathic restless legs syndrome. *Sleep.* 1999;22(7):901-12.

[5]   Taillard J, Philip P, Bioulac B. Morningness/eveningness and the need for sleep. *Journal of sleep research.* 1999;8(4):291-5.

[6]   Gangwisch JE, Feskanich D, Malaspina D, Shen S, Forman JP. Sleep duration and risk for hypertension in women: results from the nurses' health study. *American journal of hypertension.* 2013;26(7):903-11.

Chapter 2

Definition and Diagnosis

Abstract

In this chapter the reader will learn about the definition and diagnosis of Restless Legs Syndrome and Periodic Leg Movements in adults and children. The reader will also learn about the relationship between those conditions. The chapter includes an easy-to-use checklist for the healthcare professional to include in daily practice to evaluate patients afflicted by Restless Legs Syndrome and another chart to evaluate Periodic Limb Movement Disorder featuring the minimum points to diagnose the patient. The reader will learn the difference between those two conditions in diagnosis, even though they often come bound together in daily practice.

Restless Legs Syndrome Is Defined by Its Own Symptoms

Restless Legs Syndrome is a neurological condition characterized by an urge to move the legs or the arms, usually associated with paresthesia that occurs at rest and is relieved by activity [1]. The definition itself shows why physiotherapists must study and treat this condition; it is our job to relieve pain or discomfort by kinesiotherapy or other techniques available.

The symptoms strike in the evening and during the night. Several studies have shown that the severity of leg discomfort follows a circadian rhythm, with the maximum occurring after midnight [2]. The patients refer to difficulty falling asleep or waking up shortly after sleep onset with unpleasant leg sensations. They also often experience excessive daytime fatigue and somnolence as an outcome of disrupted nocturnal sleep [3], but it´s not a mandatory feature; some patients just do not have any daytime somnolence. The sensations are described as uncomfortable and unpleasant, and different terms are used such as 'ants moving' and itchy, whereas up to 59% of patients describe their sensations as painful. The pain is quite related to RLS symptoms, mainly in secondary conditions [4].

The urge to move and unpleasant leg sensations are relieved by activity (Allen et al., 2003); thus, patients use different motor strategies to relieve the discomfort. When symptoms occur, they move their legs vigorously, flexing, stretching, massaging, rubbing or crossing them one over the other. In severe cases, they walk around for hours in the evening or during the night to relieve the discomfort. The relief is usually described as beginning immediately or soon after the activity begins and it usually persists just as long as the activity continues. The worsening of symptoms in the evening or during the night is probably due to a lot of different factors. Sleep deprivation is related to worsening of the symptoms.

Another important factor is the decrease of motor activity in the evening compared with the daytime. This leads to the third possibility: the worsening of symptoms is the manifestation of an intrinsic circadian rhythm in RLS symptoms [5] that is nowadays considered a strong diagnostic feature of RLS. Recently, a symptom-provocation test called the Multiple Suggested Immobilization Test (m-sit) was validated for use in clinical trials and daily practice. It is a protocol to evaluate Periodic Leg Movements during wakefulness, the movements that relieve RLS symptoms. This test is performed several times during the day: 6:00pm, 8:00pm, 10:00pm and 12:00pm. The movements are measured in each test, every 10 minutes [6].

The severity of symptoms may fluctuate greatly throughout a patient's lifetime. During some periods, motor symptoms may be present several times a day, whereas at other times they may be totally absent. There might be sudden remissions, lasting for months or even years, without any apparent reason; these might be followed by unexplained relapses. This is one aspect targeted for future research according to the American Government [7] to ascertain how many people actually have total symptom control.

Diagnosis

The clinical diagnosis of RLS is based on the clinical evaluation of the patient. In 1995, a consensus emerged from a large International RLS Study Group (IRLSSG) on the essential criteria for the diagnosis of RLS. This group defined four clinical characteristics of RLS necessary for diagnosis (minimal criteria). These criteria were revised at a recent National Institutes of Health (NHI) RLS workshop. The final formulation of the new RLS diagnostic criteria has been published and is listed in Table 1. Patients must fulfill all the criteria [8].

Table 1. RLS criteria for adults

RLS criteria for adults	Check-list
Need to move the legs, usually associated with dysesthesia; patients may use terms like itching, tingling, pain, discomfort, irritation, anxiety and others.	Ok
Symptoms begin or increase with rest, mainly at bedtime; that characterizes the syndrome as a sleep disorder.	Ok
Relief through movement is immediate and dependent on continuous movement. Patient may need to stretch or walk. In some cases, massage or rubbing can alleviate the sensation.	Ok
Circadian pattern: it worsens on the evening or the beginning of the night, and improves late at night. It compromises the patient´s sleep until the improvement of the symptoms.	Ok
The occurrence of the abovementioned characteristics is not related to other medical or behavioral disorders (such as: myalgia, venous stasis, edema of the legs, arthritis, and leg cramps, positional discomfort, tapping the foot on the floor by habit).	Ok

In addition to these essential criteria, there are supportive clinical features that are not essential but can help resolve diagnostic uncertainty. These features include a positive family history of RLS and a positive therapeutic response to dopaminergic medications. In children the criteria for the diagnosis of RLS are different (Allen et al., 2003):

Table 2. RLS criteria for children

Child criteria	Check list		Child criteria	Check list
1. Need to move the legs, usually associated with dysesthesia; patients may use terms like itching, tingling, pain, discomfort, irritation, anxiety and others.	Ok		1. Need to move the legs, usually associated with dysesthesia; patients may use terms like itching, tingling, pain, discomfort, irritation, anxiety and others.	Ok
2. Symptoms begin or increase with rest, mainly at bedtime; this characterizes the syndrome as a sleep disorder.	Ok		2. Symptoms begin or increase with rest, mainly at bed time; this characterizes the syndrome as a sleep disorder.	Ok
3. Relief through movement is immediate and dependent on continuous movement. The patient may need to stretch or walk. In some cases, massage or rubbing can alleviate the sensation.	Ok		3. Relief through movement is immediate and dependent on continuous movement. The patient may need to stretch or walk. In some cases, massage or rubbing can alleviate the sensation.	Ok
4. Circadian pattern: it worsens in the evening or the beginning of the night, and improves late at night. It compromises the patient´s sleep until the improvement of the symptoms.	Ok	OR	4. Circadian pattern: it worsens in the evening or the beginning of the night, and improves late at night. It compromises the patient´s sleep until the improvement of the symptoms.	Ok
5. The occurrence of the abovementioned characteristics is not related to other medical or behavioral disorders (such as: myalgia, venous stasis, edema of the legs, arthritis, and leg cramps, positional discomfort, tapping the foot on the floor by habit).	Ok		5. The occurrence of the abovementioned characteristics is not related to other medical or behavioral disorders (such as: myalgia, venous stasis, edema of the legs, arthritis, and leg cramps, positional discomfort, tapping the foot on the floor by habit).	Ok
6. The child describes with his/her own words the leg discomfort.	Ok		6. Two of the three support criteria are present: a. Sleep disorder for the age	
			b. Family history	Ok
			c. Polysomnographic diagnosis of PLM	Ok

The children must meet all four of the essential diagnostic criteria established for adults, and either (1) the child must be able to describe leg discomfort in his or her own words; or (2) the child must have two of the three following features: sleep disturbance for age, A PLM index greater than 5 per hour of sleep, or a biological parent or sibling with definite RLS are supportive features [8].

Periodic Limb Movements during Sleep: The One That Comes Along in the Dark

Periodic Limb Movement (PLM) disorder is characterized by periodic episodes of repetitive and highly stereotyped limb movements that occur during sleep and by clinical sleep disturbance that cannot be accounted for by another primary sleep disorder [1]. The movements consist of extension of the big toe in combination with partial flexion of the ankle and sometimes hip. Similar movements can occur in the upper limbs. This occurrence in spinal cord injury (SCI) patients suggests the spinal origin of those movements, which could be due to the disruption of REM-related inhibitory spinal pathways producing the disconnection or disinhibition of the control pattern generator [9].

Diagnosis

It is important to discuss some introductory concepts about PLM. In some cases, the person has those movements but presents no diurnal somnolence or any other sleep disturbance symptoms. This is usually someone whose doctor finds PLM in the polysomnography checkup. It will be discussed in detail that even those cases might show autonomic activation and cardiovascular disorders in the long run. In other cases, especially those that accompany RLS, it is considered Periodic Limb Movement Disorder. The distinction between those two cases is that in the second case, the patients present symptoms of sleep disorder such as diurnal somnolence, lack of concentration or mood disorder.

The Sleep Laboratory diagnosis is based on PLM scoring. Methods for recording and scoring PLMS (periodic limb movement during sleep) were summarized by Coleman in 1982 and were revised in 2006. The diagnostic is made upon a polysomnography including electroencephalography, electrooculography, sub-mental electromyography and bilateral EMG of the anterior tibialis muscles. Experts in the field have come to a consensus to define rules for recognizing and counting limb movements. PLMS are scored only if they are part of a series of four or more consecutive movements lasting 0.5 to 5 seconds with an intermovement interval of 4 to 90 seconds. The electrographic picture of a single movement can vary from one sustained contraction to a polyclinic burst with a frequency of approximately 5 Hz. PLMS are often associated with EEG signs of arousal. PLM cluster into episodes, each of which lasts several minutes or even hours. In general, these episodes are more numerous in the first half of the night, but they can also recur throughout the entire sleep period. After recognition in the sleep study, the number of PLM per hour of sleep (PLM index) is calculated. For younger patients, a PLM index greater than 5 is considered pathological; for older patients, a PLM index greater than 15 for the entire night of sleep is considered pathological. The number of PLMS varies from night to night, especially in individuals with less severe sleep complaints [10].

In clinical researches and for clinical purposes PLM quantification is used regularly to diagnose RLS since PLM is present in 90% of RLS patients [11]. There is an important correlation between RLS, PLM and heart disease such as congestive heart failure, sympathetic activation such as alterations in pulse rate, blood pressure, systemic hypertension and even stroke [11].

PLMD has increasing importance due to possible increase in cardiovascular disorders risks, so its diagnosis is shown in Table 3 in summary according to the International Classification of Sleep Disorders [1].

It is clear that the sleep study is mandatory for PLMD diagnosis, as opposed to RLS diagnosis. The polygraphs and their software can be programed to count all the events and identify those that are PLMS clusters, but this automatic count must always be reviewed by the proper sleep lab professional. The sleep technologist must be precise in the setup of all the electrodes and other devices, so that there is minimum interference in the electrographic recordings. This precision makes it easier to identify sleep stages and all other physiological variables recorded during the sleep test. In the case of PLMD the electromyogram must be placed on the anterior tibialis correspondent area in the legs. The electroencephalogram scalp electrodes must be applied according to the International 10/20 System of Electrode Placement. The electrooculogram must be as follows: the right eye must be 1 cm lateral and 1 cm above the outside corner of the right eye, while the left eye electrode must be approximately 1 cm lateral and 1 cm below the left eye.

Table 3. Diagnostic Criteria: Periodic Limb Movement Disorder

CRITERIA	CHECK LIST
A. Insomnia or excessive sleepiness. The patient might be asymptomatic, and the movements are noticed by husband or wife or parents.	OK
B. Repetitive highly stereotyped limb muscle movements are present.	OK
C. Polysomnographic monitoring demonstrates: 1. Repetitive episodes of muscle contraction (0.5 to 5 seconds in duration) separated by an interval of typically 20 to 40 seconds; 2. Arousal or awakenings may be associated with the movements.	OK
D. The patient has no evidence of a medical or mental disorder that can account for the primary complaint.	OK
E. Other sleep disorders (e.g. obstructive sleep apnea syndrome) may be present but cannot be associated to the movements.	OK

The chin electrode placement varies from lab to lab. The respiratory effort sensors attached to belts must be placed around the chest and around the stomach. The snore sensor is placed on the neck. The airflow sensor can be either a thermistor or nasal cannula. Pressure transducers are placed under the patient's nose. The oximeter probe is placed in a finger free of nail polish [12].

All those preparations help to rule out other sleep disorders that can cause leg movements. PLMD must be differentiated from movements associated with nocturnal epileptic seizures and myoclonic epilepsy and from a number of forms of waking myoclonus, such as that seen in Lance-Adams syndrome (and tension myoclonus), Alzheimer's disease, Creutzfeldt-Jakob disease and other neuropathological conditions [1].

References

[1] American Academy of Sleep Medicine. *ICSD: International classification of sleep disorders, revised: diagnostic and coding manual.* Chicago, Illinois: American Academy of Sleep Medicine; 2001.

[2]   Síndrome das pernas inquietas: diagnóstico e tratamento. Opinião de especialistas brasileiros. *Arquivos de Neuro-Psiquiatria.* 2007;65:721-7.

[3]   Chaudhuri R, Muzerengi S. Quality of life. In: Chaudhuri R, Strambi LF, Rye D, editors. *Restless Legs Syndrome.* United States: Oxford University Press; 2008. p. 27-9.

[4]   Winkelman JW, Gagnon A, Clair AG. Sensory symptoms in restless legs syndrome: the enigma of pain. *Sleep medicine.* 2013;14(10):934-42.

[5]   Hening WA, Walters AS, Wagner M, Rosen R, Chen V, Kim S, et al. Circadian rhythm of motor restlessness and sensory symptoms in the idiopathic restless legs syndrome. *Sleep.* 1999;22(7):901-12.

[6]   Garcia-Borreguero D, Kohnen R, Boothby L, Tzonova D, Larrosa O, Dunkl E. Validation of the Multiple Suggested Immobilization Test: A Test for the Assessment of Severity of Restless Legs Syndrome (Willis-Ekbom Disease). *Sleep.* 2013;36(7):1101-9.

[7]   Carlyle M, Ouellette J, Khawaja I. Conclusions. Treatment for Restless Legs Syndrome: Future Research Needs: Identification of Future Research Needs From Comparative Effectiveness Review No 86 [Internet] United States: Agency for Healthcare Research and Quality 2013.

[8]   *Restless Legs Syndrome Foundation.* RLS Medical Bulletin2005 4/7/2012. Available from: http://www.irlssg.org/.

[9]   Telles SCL, Alves RSC, Chadi G. Periodic limb movements during sleep and restless legs syndrome in patients with ASIA A spinal cord injury. *Journal of the neurological sciences.* 2011;303(1-2):119-23.

[10] Montplaisir J, Allen RP, Walters AS, Strambi LF. Neurologic disorders. In: Kryger MH, Roth T, Dement WC, editors. *Principles and Practice of Sleep Medicine.* 5th ed. United States: Elsevier; 2011. p. 1026-37.

[11] Walters AS, Rye DB. Review of the relationship of restless legs syndrome and periodic limb movements in sleep to hypertension, heart disease, and stroke. *Sleep.* 2009;32(5):589-97.

[12] Leary E. Patient preparation. In: Butkov N, Lee-Chiong T, editors. *Fundamentals of Sleep Technology.* 1st ed. United States: Wolters Kluwer/ Lippincot Williams & Wilkins; 2007. p. 241-50.

Chapter 3

Physiopathology: Spinal Cord Theory, Dopamine Theory, Genes Related

Abstract

In this chapter the reader will read an introduction to neuroplasticity. Then the reader will learn about the physiopathology of PLM and RLS. The chapter will focus on spinal cord theory and central pattern generator, dopamine theory and the genes related to RLS and PLM. An introduction to neuroplasticity is valuable for the reader to understand all the coming chapters in the book. At the end of the chapter there will be important conclusions and remarks regarding this chapter.

Introduction to Neuroplasticity

I would like the reader to imagine a huge traffic jam. Now the reader must imagine being inside this traffic jam, tired from work and desperate to get home. The obvious decision is to try to look for another way, an empty neighborhood street that only a few people know and use, even if it is a longer and more inconvenient way. This empty street will do; it will be the way through. Our neurological system works its way through the traffic jammed areas in the superior central nervous system when there is a pathological interruption of some order. And this happens during 24 hours a day, regardless of whether the person is asleep or awake. We are also perfectly aware that when it comes to spinal cord it does not show such an ability to find other pathways. This is called neuroplasticity, the ability of our nervous system to make new connections inside our nervous system even after the first years of life, during which all of the learning process in cognitive, motor, and social behavior and their interfaces are faster and stronger for humankind.

But it is by studying the past that we might fix the present to make a better future. If the last paragraph had been read by Rene Descartes in about 1640 he would not have believed that the brain could interact with our environment at that level. According to Descartes, the sensory information would travel through the cerebrospinal fluids of our brain ventricles to get to our pineal gland, the proposed center of emotions that makes us interact with the environment in exceptional situations [1]. Now, in 2014, we are watching global efforts in brain research such as the Human Brain Project in Europe and Brain Research Through Advancing Innovative Neurotechnologies - or BRAIN in the United States. Those global efforts are based on this single subject called neuroplasticity.

Now, returning to our example: the traffic jam. When we use this example to understand a stroke, it fits perfectly to explain why some people do recover from motor paralyses using neuroplasticity in a functional outcome. But it does not explain why other people do not recover.

Using again the example of the traffic jam for chronic pain: If we as physiotherapists can teach our patients to move using different strategies, the traffic jam and alternative pathway also work perfectly, bringing the right axons to the non-painful way through neuroplasticity. But what about our patients who do not succeed?

Using the alternative street on the traffic jam model, the neurodegenerative disease would soon or later jam or destroy our alternative pathway.

It is already known by teachers that some students learn and memorize by writing, others by reading, and others by listening. So, might there be different streets in each brain for all our functions?

Return to our alternative street in the traffic jam city. Some people will find out about this empty neighborhood street in the first month, and those people will be followed by others, so that by the end of the year this street will also be jammed. This also happens in our brain. It can have a good turnout such as functional movement, or a bad turnout such as pain. So, if your alternative street is already jammed , you need to find another alternative street to get home. And so do our neurons. It is our job to manipulate and direct our axons to form the right synapses, like policemen in the traffic jam. We must understand how to show them the way. In a study resembling science fiction Pais-Vieira et al. set a brain-to-brain interaction system between rats with no other kind of communication between them. The key point is, on the sensorimotor tasks, there was a learning process in the rat receiving the information, even though this rat received no reward for his behavior at that time [2]. The explanation again is neuroplasticity.

The link between mind disorders and brain neurotransmitters has provided us with a new concept for understanding our brain perceptions. This link has been built through recent years in several Functional Magnetic Resonance (FMR) studies showing brain glucose consumption images during activities or in people afflicted by the most severe disorders, suggesting different brain patterns [3]. In RLS functional neuroimaging together with structural brain abnormalities have suggested a subcortical mechanism for RLS [4]. Spinal cord injury is followed by the action of several neurotrophic factors such as BDNF and they must be combined in such a way that the spinal cord is able to regain the ability to help with regeneration [5]. All of it must come down to how to manipulate those substances in order to help the SCI patient. This must be borne in mind: if your SCI ASIA A patient comes to you to complain about moving his feet while sleeping or restlessness in the legs in the late evening, this must be investigated. It may not be a wrong impression, hallucination or other non-explained neurological feature that our patients have because of immobilization.

In conclusion, neuroplasticity is a concept of a phenomenon that occurs in the central nervous system of a great number of living creatures, including humans. It has many ways of showing itself but it is started by a trigger strong enough to create many chemical reactions rerouting the neurons in the nervous system. Neuroplasticity is the target of possible treatments for neurological and psychiatric disorders and it is the subject of numerous scientific researches and symposiums.

1) Spinal Cord Theory and Central Pattern Generator

The central pattern generator is a structure that triggers independently, producing defense reactions or movements in animals [6]. In humans it was not tracked down anatomically, but there are numerous proofs of its presence in our spinal cord:

a) Automatic Stepping in Brain Death

Hanna and Frank [7] describe two clinical cases of automatic stepping in the pontomedullary stage of central herniation. Both cases presented large cortical infarcts leading to comatose states, and they both presented spontaneous automatic stepping, that could not be due to any external stimuli. The movements involved hip, knee and ankle, and were presented as 0.2 to 0.5 Hz bursts, lasting 5 to 45 seconds and resembling walking. According to the authors, these movements were probably due to the activation of spinal structures controlled by intact brainstem tracts. Those cases could be seen as the manifestation of mesencephalic CPG, already seen in cats [8] and also the spinal CPG.

b) Neuronal Plasticity Serving Rehabilitation

The concept that the patterns produced by spinal CPGs may have an actual function in human walking is revolutionary. But there is a huge gap from there to achieving such a goal. It seems that the simpler or less evolved the animal that produces the motor pattern the more similar it is to actual locomotion. An example in animal studies is the use of decerebrate cats that were submitted to treadmill training with electrical stimulation of an area surrounding the cuneiform nucleus [9]. The presence and absence of afferent inputs were compared. The timing of flexor and extensor muscles during locomotor activity was maintained, even though there was a higher variability without sensory input.

A very useful technique to analyze the rhythmic spinal cord activity is often applied in mice. In a study by Whelan et al. [10], the ability of the isolated lumbosacral spinal cord of the neonatal mouse to generate rhythmic motor activity has been examined. The researchers recorded spontaneous root depolarization and also evoked potentials; both had bilateral and unilateral patterns. Bath application combining N-methyl-D, L-aspartate, serotonin and dopamine also generated rhythmic alternate locomotor-like movements. They also proved that reciprocal inhibitory connections between the left and right sides of the cord are not essential for the rhythmic pattern, for those were preserved following the mid-sagittal section of the spinal cord.

The maturation of human gait may involve reorganization in the spinal circuitry and more extensive supraespinal dependency in the regulation of locomotion than in lower vertebrates [11, 12]. So it is quite a challenge, so far unbeaten, to manipulate human CPG for rehabilitation.

Another important factor is the usefulness of this manipulation. The balance needed for walking comes from supraespinal influences, and even if the CPG was reconnected, it would not by itself make a regular standard walking pattern in a SCI patient.

There have been recent studies that show how neuroplasticity is being used in SCI rehabilitation. The most used techniques are treadmill walking and robotics. None of those include the American Spinal Injury Association (ASIA) A patients [13-15].

One single-blind randomized trial by Dobkin et al. [15] entered for rehabilitation 107 ASIA C and D patients and 38 B patients with recent lesions between C5 and L3 who were unable to walk on admission. The trial compared 12 weeks of step-training with body-weight support on a treadmill with overground practice to a more conventional intervention. Their conclusions were that few ASIA B and most ASIA C and D patients achieved functional walking ability by the end of 12 weeks of treadmill walking training protocol. Another interesting conclusion is that walking-related measures assessed at 2-week intervals revealed that the length of time after SCI is an important variable for entering patients into a trial with mobility outcomes. This means that the faster the patient starts this training protocol, the better functional results he or she might have.

Another study by Dobkin et al. [14] compared the efficacy of step training with body weight support on a treadmill (BWSTT) with over-ground practice to the efficacy of a defined over-ground mobility therapy (CONT). 146 subjects, graded on ASIA as B, C, or D with levels from C5 to L3, from six regional centers within 8 weeks of SCI were entered in a single-blind, multicenter, randomized clinical trial. They received 12 weeks of equal time of BWSTT or CONT. No significant differences were found at entry or at 6 months for Functional Independence Measure Locomotion (n=108) and walking speed and distance (n=72). The conclusions were that the physical therapy strategies of body weight support on a treadmill and defined overground mobility therapy did not produce different outcomes. This finding was partly due to the unexpectedly high percentage of ASIA C subjects who achieved functional walking speeds, irrespective of treatment.

Another interesting study [16] compares the metabolic costs during robotic and therapist-assisted treadmill walking in 10 individuals with incomplete spinal cord injury. Metabolic and electromyographic (EMG) data were collected during standing and stepping on the treadmill in both cases. During robotic-assisted walking, subjects were asked to match the kinematic trajectories of the device and maximize their effort. During therapist-assisted walking, subjects walked on the treadmill with manual assistance provided as necessary. Their results were significantly lower metabolic costs and lower swing-phase hip flexor EMG activity, when subjects were asked to match the robotic device trajectories, than with therapist-assisted walking. These differences were reduced when subjects were asked to maximize their effort during robotic-assisted stepping, although swing-phase plantar-flexor EMG activity was increased. In addition, during standing prior to therapist- or robotic-assisted stepping, metabolic costs were higher without stabilization from the robotic device.

c) Flexor Referent Afferent and the Central Pattern Generator

The Flexor Referent Afferent (FRA) would be the tool through which the spinal CPG would act. Paulus et al. [17] proposed that FRA would be responsible for PLM and for the relief caused by movement in RLS. They also propose that FRA would be responsible for more complex movements during sleep.

d) Animal Models for PLM

Another promising mean of studying the neuronal connections that lie within the spinal cord affected by PLM would be by using animal models. Ondo et al. [18] reviewed animal models for RLS and PLM based on iron deprivation and destruction of the A11 diencephalic spinal tract. They discuss specifically for RLS 6-hydroxydopamine lesioned rat model with and without iron deficiency and also dopamine D3 receptor knockout mice. For PLM they discuss the effect of haloperidol, a dopamine antagonist, in rats. Their conclusions are that even though the RLS animal models might help to find out more about the involvement of dopaminergic action or iron depletion in the syndrome, it's not a perfect model since it comes without the clinical sensory components that characterize the syndrome in humans. One interesting point is that PLM is seen as a behavioral marker for RLS in animal models, so those models might be closer to human PLM itself than for human RLS.

Following the idea of studying PLM for itself, Esteves et al. [19] describe a mouse animal model in 10 rats submitted to T9 lesions. There were four different types of lesion: Group 0 with no hystopathological alterations (SHAM group), Group I: predominantly affecting central part of dorsal column, Group II: predominantly affecting the entire dorsal column, Group III: affecting mainly the hemimedula, including the whole dorsal column and Group IV: almost all the spinal cord. Their results showed that 10 out of 11 rats presented limb movements during sleep, while the SHAM group presented no limb movements during the experiment. Their conclusions are that these movements are probably generated by a spinal CPG, without the involvement of cortical inputs. This model brings us another concept which is to find the spinal mechanisms responsible for PLM, but those kinds of studies are quite rare.

In humans, there are major controversies with regard to the localization of the neural structures involved in the physiopathological process of RLS, but there is most likely a major contribution of the spinal cord. Bara-Jimenez et al. [20] studied the flexion reflex of patients with primary RLS by electrically stimulating the plantar nerve. They found a facilitation of the late component of flexor reflex afferent, indicating hyperexcitability of motoneurons in this condition. They also noted that the late components shared several features with PLMS. Those studies suggest the presence of a spinal cord generator for the periodic motor manifestations of RLS. This spinal cord generator might be facilitated by the suppression of or decrease in supraespinal inhibitory inputs.

2) Genes Related to PLM and RLS

This part will be reviewed but the materials and methods applied by the geneticists are beyond the scope of this book.

The importance of the discovery and mapping of genes in RLS and PLM was definitive for the recognition and respect for those afflicted by these conditions. Before this discovery many used to say that RLS simply did not exist. There might be many colleagues in healthcare in other countries who have never heard about this condition. But here it is, mapped and proven to be a condition affecting humans.

Genetic Heterogeneity of Restless Legs Syndrome (OMIM 102300)

RLS1 has been mapped to chromosome 12q. Other susceptibility loci for RLS include RLS2 (608831) on chromosome 14q13-q31; RLS3 (610438) on chromosome 9p24-p22; RLS4 (610439) on chromosome 2q33; RLS5 (611242) on chromosome 20p13; RLS6 (611185) on chromosome 6p21; RLS7 (612853) on chromosome 2p14; and RLS8 (615197) on chromosome 5q31. The several phenotypes could be justified by the repetition of those single nucleotide polymorphisms or by the presence of more genes already mapped to RLS in humans.

There might be entire families affected by RLS, or even different generations. A study was conducted involving 300 RLS patients; 232 of whom were considered idiopathic and the others were secondary to uremia. The authors observed a definite family history of RLS, defined as at least 1 first-degree relative with verified RLS, in 42% of idiopathic RLS patients and, surprisingly, 12% of patients with RLS secondary to uremia. [21].

There is strong evidence suggesting a hereditary component in PLM. A recent article showed an association between a sequence variant in chromosome 6p and PLM in distinct Icelandic and American cohorts of subjects with RLS and their families [22].

A simultaneous report by [23] showed an association between the same sequence variant and two additional single nucleotide polymorphisms in German and Canadian cohorts with RLS. Thus, PLM would serve as a heritable biological marker or endophenotype for RLS.

Then, we as physiotherapists would face the reasonable and quite mandatory question: do our SCI patients have those genes? Reviewing the genetic studies I have not found researches regarding SCI, RLS and related genes. If they do have them, would those genes trigger and manifest themselves after - or because of - the spinal cord injury?

Conclusion and Remarks

It is quite important to summarize key points to connect them to the following chapters:

- RLS is a real chronic neurological disturbance in all aspects: standard presentation in idiopathic and secondary cases showing mapped genes
- RLS is linked to PLM in a most definite way. Neither has been understood in its physiopathology
- As a chronic disorder, like many we handle as physiotherapists in our daily clinic, it will come in the natural history of stronger or lighter symptoms. Those triggers will be thoroughly discussed in the following chapters even though they are not yet fully understood
- In all hypotheses, neuroplasticity appears as a decisive factor and must accompany all the clinical decisions involving RLS in all health professionals' daily clinics

References

[1]   René Descartes: Wikipedia; 2013 [updated 12/21/2013; cited 2013 12/22/2013]. Contents [hide].

[2]   Pais-Vieira M, Lebedev M, Kunicki C, Wang J, Nicolelis MA. A brain-to-brain interface for real-time sharing of sensorimotor information. *Scientific reports.* 2013;3:1319.

[3]   Brewer JA, Garrison KA, Whitfield-Gabrieli S. What about the "Self" is Processed in the Posterior Cingulate Cortex? *Frontiers in human neuroscience.* 2013;7:647.

[4]   Desseilles M, Dang-Vu T, Schabus M, Sterpenich V, Maquet P, Schwartz S. Neuroimaging insights into the pathophysiology of sleep disorders. *Sleep.* 2008;31(6):777-94.

[5]   McCall J, Weidner N, Blesch A. Neurotrophic factors in combinatorial approaches for spinal cord regeneration. *Cell and tissue research.* 2012;349(1):27-37.

[6]   Telles SC, Alves RS, Chadi G. Spinal cord injury as a trigger to develop periodic leg movements during sleep: an evolutionary perspective. *Arquivos de neuro-psiquiatria.* 2012;70(11):880-4.

[7]   Hanna JP, Frank JI. Automatic stepping in the pontomedullary stage of central herniation. *Neurology.* 1995;45(5):985-6.

[8]   Vinay L, Padel Y, Bourbonnais D, Steffens H. An ascending spinal pathway transmitting a central rhythmic pattern to the magnocellular red nucleus in the cat. *Exp Brain Res.* 1993;97(1):61-70.

[9]   Grillner S, Zangger P. The effect of dorsal root transection on the efferent motor pattern in the cat's hindlimb during locomotion. *Acta Physiol Scand.* 1984;120(3):393-405.

[10] Whelan P, Bonnot A, O'Donovan MJ. Properties of rhythmic activity generated by the isolated spinal cord of the neonatal mouse. *J Neurophysiol.* 2000;84(6):2821-33.

[11] Forrsberg H, Hirchsfield H, Stokes VP. Developments of Human Locomotion mechanisms. In: Shimamura M. GS, Edgerton V.R., editor. *Neurobiological Basis of Human Locomotion.* Tokyo, Japan: Japan Scientif Society Press; 1991. p. 259-73.

[12] MacKay-Lyons M. Central pattern generation of locomotion: a review of the evidence. *Phys Ther.* 2002;82(1):69-83.

[13] Alcobendas-Maestro M, Lopez-Dolado E, Esclarin de Ruz A, Valdizan-Valledor MC. [Gait training in incomplete spinal cord injuries with body weight support]. *Rev Neurol.* 2004;39(5):406-10.

[14] Dobkin B, Apple D, Barbeau H, Basso M, Behrman A, Deforge D, et al. Weight-supported treadmill vs over-ground training for walking after acute incomplete SCI. *Neurology.* 2006;66(4):484-93.

[15] Dobkin B, Barbeau H, Deforge D, Ditunno J, Elashoff R, Apple D, et al. The evolution of walking-related outcomes over the first 12 weeks of rehabilitation for incomplete traumatic spinal cord injury: the multicenter randomized Spinal Cord Injury Locomotor Trial. *Neurorehabil Neural Repair.* 2007;21(1):25-35.

[16] Israel JF, Campbell DD, Kahn JH, Hornby TG. Metabolic costs and muscle activity patterns during robotic- and therapist-assisted treadmill walking in individuals with incomplete spinal cord injury. *Phys Ther.* 2006;86(11):1466-78.

[17] Paulus W, Schomburg ED. Dopamine and the spinal cord in restless legs syndrome: does spinal cord physiology reveal a basis for augmentation? *Sleep medicine reviews.* 2006;10(3):185-96.

[18] Ondo WG, Zhao HR, Le WD. Animal models of restless legs syndrome. *Sleep medicine.* 2007;8(4):344-8.

[19] Esteves AM, de Mello MT, Lancellotti CL, Natal CL, Tufik S. Occurrence of limb movement during sleep in rats with spinal cord injury. *Brain Res.* 2004;1017(1-2):32-8.

[20] Bara-Jimenez W, Aksu M, Graham B, Sato S, Hallett M. Periodic limb movements in sleep: state-dependent excitability of the spinal flexor reflex. *Neurology.* 2000;54(8):1609-16.

[21] Winkelmann J, Czamara D, Schormair B, Knauf F, Schulte EC, Trenkwalder C, et al. Genome-wide association study identifies novel restless legs syndrome susceptibility loci on 2p14 and 16q12.1. *PLoS genetics.* 2011;7(7):e1002171.

[22] Stefansson H, Rye DB, Hicks A, Petursson H, Ingason A, Thorgeirsson TE, et al. A genetic risk factor for periodic limb movements in sleep. *N Engl J Med.* 2007;357(7):639-47.

[23] Winkelman JW. Periodic Limb Movements in Sleep -- Endophenotype for Restless Legs Syndrome? *N Engl J Med.* 2007.

Chapter 4

Related Diseases and Conditions in Physiotherapy Practice

Abstract

In this chapter the discussion deepens within the main topic of the book. The reader will learn about the epidemiology of SCI related to RLS and PLM. The neurotransmitter dysfunctions including dopaminergic agents, iron and opioid texts will bring the reader closer to the discussions that surround the congress and scientific discussions regarding RLS and PLM. The treatment of SCI patients proposed in the literature will be detailed and discussed, focusing on exercise for idiopathic cases. The diagnosis and handling of RLS in amputees follows the discussion of this specific physiopathological condition. Finally, the impressive overlap of RLS and fibromyalgia will be discussed along with the importance of handling the sleep disorder in such a patient for a more effective outcome in physiotherapy rehabilitation.

Introduction

The prevalence of PLM in the population is 3.9% [1]. There are several genes related to the disorder transmission [2].

The RLS has clinical diagnosis; therefore, the prevalence and incidence may vary according to the study criteria. If only the symptoms are considered, the prevalence varies from 9.4% to 15%. If the minimum diagnostic criteria from the International Restless Leg Syndrome Study Group [1], are considered, the prevalence varies from 3.9% to 14.3%. When factors like severity and frequency are taken in consideration, the prevalence varies from 2.2% to 7.9%. When performing the differential diagnostic procedure, the prevalence varies from 1.9% to 4.6%. The prevalence is higher in women and increases with age [3].

There are other medical conditions to which RLS and PLM have been related. RLS is often associated with uremia that can be prevalent in 25.3% of end-stage renal disease patients according to a large multicenter study performed in Taiwan on 1130 patients [4]. There is some evidence suggesting an association between RLS and peripheral neuropathy: it can be present in 44% of diabetics afflicted by peripheral neuropathy [5]. A relationship between RLS and iron and folic-acid deficient anemia has also been reported [4]. Also, RLS was found in 64% of 332 female patients with fibromyalgia [6]. In addition, several medications and other substances may induce or worsen RLS or PLMS. These include tricyclic or other antidepressants, lithium carbonate, dopamine D2 receptor blocking agents, such as neuroleptics, as well as alcohol [7].

PLMS should be differentiated from other state-dependent motor disorders such as sleep-related "myoclonus", also called hypnic myoclonus or "sleep starts"; "painful legs and moving toes" syndrome; nocturnal leg cramps; neuroleptic-induced akathisia; vascular conditions such as vascular or neurogenic intermittent claudication are frequent causes of leg pain or discomfort, but have different clinical signs compared to RLS.

In doubtful diagnosis the medical investigation should include two consecutive nights of polysomnographic recordings; a careful clinical examination of sensory and motor functions should be performed and EMG and nerve conduction studies should be performed if the examination suggests peripheral neuropathy or radiculopathy. Also, iron status should be studied in every patient with standard serum tests for ferritin; total iron-biding capacity, and percentage saturation should be considered an essential part of the clinical examination.

Periodic Limb Movement (PLM) disorder is characterized by periodic episodes of repetitive and highly stereotyped limb movements that occur during sleep. The movements usually occur in the legs and consist of extension of the big toe in combination with partial flexion of the ankle, and sometimes the hip. Similar movements can occur in the upper limbs [8]. This occurrence in spinal cord injured (SCI) patients leads toward the theory that proposes the spinal origin of those movements, which could be due to the disruption of REM-related inhibitory spinal pathways producing the disconnection or disinhibition of a spinal generator or pacemaker [9].

SCI, PLM and RLS

Epidemiology

Spinal cord injury patients presenting PLM are quite rare. One article discussed a single case showing the disconnections between those movements and the cortical arousals [10].

In my research analyzing SCI our group evaluated 24 subjects: The Control Group (CG) was composed of 16 subjects, 50% of each sex. The Spinal Cord Injury Group (SCIG) was composed of 8 subjects with complete SCI, 100% male (p=0.02), with 3.61 ± 1.72 years of injury time. CG subjects were 24.38 ± 4.03 years of age while SCIG subjects were 29 ± 5.21 years old (p=0.02). Those patients were submitted to a full night's polysomnography and were assessed using the Epworth Sleepiness Scale and an adapted form of International Restless Legs Syndrome Scale Score. 100% of subjects from SCIG presented RLS compared to 17% in CG (p < 0.0001). SCIG had 18.11±20.07 of PLM index while CG had 5.96 ± 11.93 (p=0.01). There was a positive moderate correlation between RLS and age (r=0.5; p=0.01) RLS and PLM (r=0.49; p=0.01), adapted International Restless Legs Syndrome rating scale and PLM index (r=0.64; p=0.03) and a negative moderate correlation between the Epworth Sleepiness Scale and PLM index (r=-0.4; p=0.04).

Since the first neural CPG theory proposed by Graham Brown through his experiments on cats [11], the most compelling evidence of human CPG is the occurrence of PLM in SCI patients. This model of CPG is a simple model: when one neurone (half-center) is activated it depresses the other synchronously with the activation of its own effector. But that other "half-center" when active depresses the first, and when it is depressed its depression of the first half–center is diminished in value. Therefore, the activation of the first will increase still further. He called this progressive augmentation of activation by the process of mutual inhibition. Applying this theory to the SCI patients and PLM is quite admissible but there is a lack of evidence. The few studies available are mostly case discussion and the human CPG has not been located or activated in the same way that it has in cats [12]. Mello et al. [13]

verified the prevalence of sleep complaints in SCI patients, characterized by a complete section.

There are many other theories regarding PLM in SCI patients that have been presented but little evidence to support them. In summary, it is not known whether PLM would be a consequence of the absence of superior efferences to the spinal cord, which would cause an increase in the excitability of the motoneurons, or if it is a primary phenomenon coming from an alleged generator located inside the human spinal cord. If its origin is in the superior central nervous system, it is not known if PLM would correlate with the sleep stage [9], relative concentration of iron in the red nucleus [14], lack of iron in the blood caused by anemia, or central neurotransmitter disorders [12]. If its origin is intrinsic to the spinal cord, the action of the neurotransmitters in the spinal cord might be one of the causes of PLM.

Whenever there is an SCI injury, it is accompanied by many neurological features that characterize SCI injuries such as alterations in tonus, muscular strength, sensibility and others. The reader must remember that those neurological alterations are in fact due to the level of injury in the spinal cord and are dependent upon whether it was a complete or incomplete injury. Those are neuroplasticity related events which - as in brain injuries - lead to the deterioration of neurological function. Possibly, in those cases, PLM is a manifestation of the release of the spinal generator, resulting in leg movements.

Neurotransmitter Dysfunctions

Several new studies suggest the involvement of the dopamine system and depletion of iron stores in RLS. PLM may be related to dopamine deficiency; it is more common in conditions with dopamine deficiency and less common in conditions with dopamine excess. Therapeutic results obtained with opioids and L-dopa have led to some neuropharmacological hypotheses regarding the physiopathological process of RLS-PLM.

1. Dopaminergic Agents

The Practice Parameters for the Dopaminergic Treatment of RLS and PLM [15], after the effectiveness of levodopa with decarboxylase inhibitor, dopamine agonist pergolide, dopamine agonist pramipexole and dopamine agonist ropinirole. Other dopamine agonists are not certified, such as the dopaminergic agents amantadine and selegine. The EFNS guidelines on the management of Restless Legs Syndrome and Periodic Leg Movements in sleep [16], also analyzed several dopaminergic agents: for primary RLS levodopa is effective in the short term and probably effective in the long term follow-up; in the short term there were minor side effects, while in the long term there was a 30-70% drop out due to adverse effects or lack of efficacy. Augmentation occurred in 20-92% of the patients.

A very interesting point of view can be read in a theoretical review [17], in which the authors conceal the physiology of the spinal cord to better explain the phenomenon of augmentation. It would be caused by a second-delayed action of L-DOPA, which would consist of facilitation of long-latency FRA pathways and an introduction of rhythmic movements. Dopamine is a movement related neurotransmitter. Interestingly, physical exercise might reduce PLM in SCI patients [18]: the study involved acute and chronic exercise. The acute intensive exercise group consisted of 22 volunteers who underwent a maximum effort test and a polysomnography (PSG) on the same night. The chronic exercise group included 11 patients who performed 72 physical training sessions undergoing three PSG studies on the night of sessions 1, 36, and 72.

Both forms of physical exercise lowered PLM levels. The acute physical exercise increased sleep efficiency, rapid eye movement (REM) sleep, and reduced wake after sleep onset, whereas the chronic physical exercise increased sleep efficiency, REM sleep, and reduced sleep latency. A good explanation for this phenomenon could be that somehow physical exercise would inhibit some pathway connected to FRA reflexes which by consequence would no longer be so excited and would elicit fewer rhythmic movements.

The EFNS guidelines on the management of Restless Legs Syndrome and Periodic Leg Movements in sleep [16] analyzed more dopaminergic agents that were classified as ergot and non-ergot derivatives. The ergot derivatives are α-dihydroergocryptine, bromocriptine, carbegoline, lisuride, pergolide and terguride. The non-ergot derivatives are pramipexole, ropinirole and rotigotine. For the ergot-derivatives, α-dihydroergocryptine, lisuride and terguride have not yet been studied in a high class of evidence studies, so there is not enough evidence about their effectiveness. For primary RLS, there was a double-blind randomized crossover trial comparing pergolide and levodopa which pointed out the better outcome with pergolide treatment in 82% of patients when compared with 9% levodopa; more than that, pergolide caused a

79% reduction in the PLMS index when compared with 45% of levodopa [19]. But pergolide is probably ineffective in RLS secondary to uremia [16]. Cabergoline is also effective in the short term and possibly effective in long-term follow-up for primary RLS. There was a recent random large-scale double-blind study of two active dopaminergic therapies for Restless Legs Syndrome [20], the dopamine agonist cabergoline and levodopa/benserazide (levodopa). Patients with idiopathic RLS were treated with fixed daily doses of 2 or 3 mg of cabergoline or 200 or 300 mg of levodopa for 30 weeks. More patients in the levodopa group (24.0%) than in the cabergoline group discontinued because of loss of efficacy. This first large-scale active controlled study in RLS showed the superior efficacy of cabergoline versus levodopa after a 30-week trial [21].

Regarding the non-ergot derivatives, ropinirole was the most extensively studied drug, being considered effective for primary RLS [16] and also producing significant benefits on objective measures of RLS motor symptoms, such as Periodic Leg Movements, and subjective measures of sleep [22]. Rotigotine by transdermal patch-delivery is effective [23]. Rotigotine transdermal patches releasing 2 to 3 mg/24 hr significantly reduced the severity of RLS symptoms. Treatment efficacy was maintained throughout the 6-month double-blind period.

Regarding pramipexole, it is probably effective in short-term follow-up [16]. Recently there was a study of the long-term efficacy and safety of pramipexole in patients with RLS [24]. They found the most frequent side effects include influenza (17.8%), headache (15.0%), and fatigue (10.3%). Their conclusion is that pramipexole is well tolerated and effective for the long-term treatment of RLS.

The therapeutic effects of L-dopa and dopaminergic agonists on RLS and PLMS support the hypothesis that central dopamine may be involved in the pathophysiology of these conditions. Brain imaging studies have been inconsistent.

One study showed small but significant decreased striatal binding for raclopride, suggesting either decreased D2 receptor activity or increased intracellular dopamine, or both [25]. Prior studies using positron emission tomography (PET) or single-photon emission computed tomography techniques have reported inconsistent findings regarding the differences between patients with Restless Legs Syndrome [20] and control patients in the striatal dopamine-2 receptor (D2R) binding potentials (BP).Thirty-one patients with primary RLS and 36 age- and sex-matched control patients completed the study. They found increased synaptic putamen dopamine in putamen [26].

2. Iron

Along with dopamine, there is evidence that iron may also be important in Restless Legs Syndrome. Conditions such as iron-deficient anemia, end-stage renal disease and pregnancy have been clearly established as causes of secondary RLS [12]. All of these conditions involve iron deficiency. Yet it's still not known how iron interacts with dopamine in such a way as to change the pathology of Restless Legs Syndrome [12]. Cho et al. [27] conducted a study in which idiopathic RLS patients drawn from the Korean population received four weekly intravenous (IV) doses of 250 mg low-molecular weight iron dextran for a total dose of 1g. One week after the last dose, any subject on RLS medication tapered off the RLS medications. Blood and CSF samples were taken to measure iron parameters at baseline and again three weeks after the last dose. Twenty-five patients (age 55.2 ± 9.3, 18 female) enrolled in this study without serious adverse reactions. Seventeen of the 25 patients (68%) showed moderate or complete improvement of all RLS symptoms after treatment based on the Korean-translated versions of the International RLS Severity scale (K-IRLS). Changes in the K-IRLS did not correlate significantly with changes in CSF ferritin. The response to IV iron could not be predicted from patients' demographics, or by blood or CSF iron baseline characteristics. RLS symptom improvement started between one and six weeks after treatment and the treatment benefits lasted from one month to 22 months. Fourteen patients (56%) completely stopped all medications, for a mean duration of 31.3 ± 33.1 weeks. These results are comparable to those from a prior study with high molecular weight dextran, which according to the authors is more dangerous than the low molecular weight dextran.

3. Opioids

The same assumption might be made concerning opioids, since it is an efficient treatment in RLS. But so far the exact mechanism of action by which opioids improves the symptoms is not known [12]. A recent study investigated the efficacy and safety of a combination of oxycodone-naloxone for patients whose treatment was not successful with previous drugs. It was a multicenter study consisting of a 12-week randomized, double-blind, placebo-controlled trial and 40-week open-label extension phase done at 55 sites in Austria, Germany, Spain, and Sweden. Patients had symptoms for at least 6 months and an International RLS Study Group severity rating scale sum score of at least 15; patients with severe chronic obstructive pulmonary disease or a history of sleep apnea syndrome were excluded. The study drug was oxycodone 5·0 mg, naloxone 2·5 mg, twice per day, which was up-titrated according to the investigator's opinion to a maximum of oxycodone 40 mg, naloxone 20 mg, twice per day; in the extension, all patients started on oxycodone 5·0 mg, naloxone 2·5 mg, twice per day, which was up-titrated to a maximum of oxycodone 40 mg, naloxone 20 mg, twice per day. The primary outcome was a mean change in the severity of symptoms according to the International RLS Study Group severity rating scale sum score at 12 weeks. 495 patients were evaluated, of whom 306 were randomly assigned and 276 included in the primary analysis (132 to prolonged release oxycodone-naloxone vs 144 to placebo). 197 patients participated in the open-label extension. The mean International RLS Study Group rating scale sum score at randomization was 31·6 (SD 4·5); the mean change after 12 weeks was -16·5 (SD 11·3) in the prolonged release oxycodone-naloxone group and -9·4 (SD 10·9) in the placebo group (the mean difference between groups at 12 weeks was 8·15, 95% CI 5·46-10·85; p<0·0001).

After the extension phase, the mean sum score was 9·7 (SD 7·8). Treatment-related adverse events occurred in 109 of 150 (73%) patients in the prolonged release oxycodone-naloxone group and 66 of 154 (43%) in the placebo group during the double-blind phase; during the extension phase, 112 of 197 (57%) had treatment-related adverse events. Five of 306 (2%) patients had serious treatment-related adverse events when taking prolonged release oxycodone-naloxone (vomiting with concurrent duodenal ulcer, constipation, subileus, ileus, acute flank pain). The conclusion was that the combination of oxycodone and naloxone was effective in short-term treatment [28].

Treatment of SCI Patients Afflicted by RLS and PLM

It is important to clarify a concept. The patients discussed here had different etiologies and degrees of SCI. The physiotherapist has an important intervention in all of those patients alike. If the etiology is an accident and it is a complete or ASIA A SCI, the prognosis of movement recovery is very narrow, as opposed to other kinds of SCI. The physiotherapist must bear in mind the fact that - regardless of the etiology of the SCI - this event might trigger the RLS or PLMD.

Salminen et al. [10] reported a case of a SCI patient treated for sleep apnea, yet still presenting PLMS. Afterwards, the movements were suppressed by pramipexole. By analyzing those movements and microarousals, they found no temporal connection between those two phenomena, as expected. According to the authors, the disconnection of PLMs from arousals supports a spinal generator or peripheral trigger mechanism for PLMs. The suppression of movements by a dopamine agonist suggests that its site of action is caudal to the cervical lesion. Those conclusions are based on animal models and a diencephalic tract that connects is A11 to the spinal cord in rats. This animal model was discussed in depth in the study of Clemens et al. [29] in which D3 receptors were found to play the leading role in the rat spinal cord transmitting nervous potentials to trigger PLM.

Nilsonn et al. [30] reported the RLS symptoms in four SCI patients. According to the text they were misdiagnosed and were considered refractory cases of neuropathic pain. One of them had an ASIA A injury. They were all treated with pramipexole.

To reinforce the theory that virtually any spinal cord damage might trigger RLS, Irkec et al. [31] describe a multiple sclerosis case with sudden onset of RLS symptoms. The reader must note that it is a case that involves the spinal cord.

Lee et al. [32] reported SCI due to a schwannoma in one patient and intramedullary lesions in two others. They were cases of thoracic injury. The authors suggest that those lesions partially disinhibited the lumbosacral generator.

There has already been a study that compares physical exercise and L-DOPA in SCI patients. A total of 13 volunteers received L-DOPA (200 mg) and benserazide (50 mg) 1 h before sleeping for 30 days and were then submitted to a physical exercise program on a manual bicycle ergometer for 45 days (3 times a week). Both L-DOPA administration (35.11-19.87 PLM/h, $P<0.03$) and physical exercise (35.11-18.53 PLM/h, $P<0.012$) significantly reduced PLM; however, no significant difference was observed between the two types of treatment [33].

All those evidences are extremely important for our daily practice, but the most important result is that exercise has a potential benefit for those patients. We should be careful according to what has already been the topic of discussion in this book: the few scientific evidences provided for exercise in this kind of patient do not necessarily mean that this intervention does not work. The problem is that the double-blind placebo methodology used for medications does not apply for exercise, as the patient will know if he is doing the exercise or not. That is a barrier for other researchers to avoid publishing papers in this kind of topic. But the exercises did decrease PLM index in PSG, which is a concrete result. They might, in my opinion, help decrease RLS symptoms if that is the case.

Quite on time, there are researchers who recognize the importance of exercise and non-drug therapies for RLS. One paper by Mitchell [34] reviews non-drug therapies including exercise and even massage and NIR light that are the daily practice of physiotherapists. All those therapies have unknown physiological mechanisms that justify their effectiveness, just like many other drugs used for this condition.

To implement an exercise program the physiotherapist must show, other than evidence, the cost effectiveness of the intervention to the healthcare industry. A number of studies are available in the literature and are discussed here to show examples. Depending on the location and country, the healthcare system is different and the results might be different. Davis et al. [35] report a comparison between three kinds of exercise: aerobic, tonus and balance or resistance training for patients afflicted by mild cognitive impairment. It was a public health study that lasted six months with classes twice a week. They found that aerobic and resistance training was more cost-effective than balance training for this pathology. To reach this conclusion they collected information about healthcare program use, used the stroop test to analyze cognitive features in 6 months, and based their cohort in previous epidemiology studies.

In the case of RLS, the tool to analyze the improvement is usually the RLS scale, but quality of life indicators are also very important regarding healthcare politics, mainly dealing with RLS that is chronic and incurable.

Also physical exercise and non-drug therapies have inbuilt safety if appropriately applied by a qualified physiotherapist. This is a universal fact regardless of the location.

Also, RLS medical doctors are not available everywhere. On the other hand, for example, in Brazil by April 2013 there were 176.176 registered physiotherapists in the country which has a population of almost 200,000,000, about 5% of which might be affected by RLS given our mixture of European and African origins; 10,000,000 is a good estimate of the number of people afflicted by this disorder in Brazil. To follow up a prescribed drug therapy it requires a medical doctor who is an expert in sleep disorder. To manage an aerobic exercise routine it requires a non-specialist physiotherapist.

You can apply this math for your location seeking information in your Physiotherapy Official organization or in Public Health Care organizations.

The challenge of implementing exercise as a treatment for an incurable condition such as RLS is that any musculoskeletal condition might impair the participation of the subject in the exercise program. The general health professional has limited resources to handle this condition, but the physiotherapist can adapt the exercise program promptly and obviously treat the musculoskeletal condition depending on its severity, in the short or long term.

As a conclusion to this topic which is fundamental to this book, we can say that exercise is a cost-effective intervention for RLS patients, including SCI patients. In this last case, an adapted bicycle is necessary. Those are safe interventions that improve RLS symptoms though improving the quality of life. This kind of intervention does not require a medical doctor who is an expert in RLS, although the presence of this professional would be a precious acquisition for such a group. To treat such an unknown disorder accordingly, it would be advisable to also implement an education program in your community. This disorder is often not recognized and rarely heard of. Exercise and physiotherapy are not valued or recognized as an effective intervention by many patients. In my daily practice, the patients (regardless of their pathology) describe physiotherapy in general as "palliative", "not worth the effort", "not worth coming" and other similar expressions. The way to change this is through the explanation and education of the patient and the family to keep the adhesion to the program whatever resource you are using in your consultation.

Finally, we must not lose sight of the neuroplasticity that exercise intervention might bring to our patients. This is especially true for SCI, but also important for all kinds of RLS patients. There have been no studies regarding changes in SCI neuroplasticity before and after a program of physical exercise regarding the RLS symptoms. But there might be a hypothesis since there is improvement in SCI sequels following rehabilitation programs. This hypothesis in itself is a strong reason to implement an exercise protocol for those patients.

Amputation and Restless Legs Syndrome: Physiopathology Theories, Phantom Pain, Possible Interventions

As I was studying the amazing facts found during my research, I came across something that would seem even more surreal to non-scholars or researchers - the presence of RLS symptoms in amputees [36]. This was followed by some case studies [37] that responded to dopaminergic medication.

As physiotherapists we must know how to deal with RLS in amputees. This large cohort [36] that found RLS symptoms evaluated several causes of limb loss: trauma, vascular disease, cancer, infection, gangrene, diabetes with or without vascular disease, congenital limb deficiency and correction cases, toxic shock syndrome, Charcot-Marie Tooth, rheumatoid arthritis, polio and Dupuytren´s contracture. The classic phantom sensations were divided into categories of non-painful, phantom pain and both, and were present respectively in 73.14%, 67.5% and both 47.7%. Of this population, 13% reported RLS phantom pain. The cases that were treated with dopaminergic medication raised discussions in the paper. The neuropathy also raised discussions and it is important that the physiotherapist is aware of that correlation. The central regions that compensate in brain maps are quite classical in the neurology of the amputee and are expected in all amputees. The presence or absence of RLS symptoms cannot be appointed as a major cause of such a brain change.

This book is filled with examples of the spinal cord acting in RLS, so the presence of RLS symptoms in amputees is another evidence of the spinal generator in those symptoms. Other diencephalic alterations in neural transmissions may be present, but in amputees it is more likely that the undressing of the stump in the evening triggers peripherical nervous stimulation to the point that it has to be rubbed or hit. The patient response in the case described is exactly what a SCI patient reported in the interview I performed. It was really hitting hard his methodology of surpassing RLS symptoms.

This book was also written with the aim of clarifying that we have passed the phase of amazing neurology discoveries and are entering the phase of dealing with those patients. The more physiotherapists are aware of the presence of RLS symptoms in amputees, the faster we might come up with a treatment for those patients. Up to now, the dopaminergic medications are the only possible intervention, so more researchers in our field are necessary to unravel the amputee phantom pain.

Fibromyalgia and Restless Legs Syndrome: Physiopathology and Role of Physical Therapy

Fibromyalgia has an unknown cause and manifests itself through pain and compromising the quality of life. It has a huge prevalence since it permeates among a very productive age range and generates great social-economic impact. Physiotherapy has an important role in its treatment and control of the symptoms. Therapeutic exercises are being postulated as one of the main tools in the management of FM with solid scientific evidence, including the sleep disturbances patients also present.

Fibromyalgia has an important overlap with RLS. It is also known that fibromyalgia patients present sleep disorders. To start to understand the possible connection the reader must follow Figure 1:

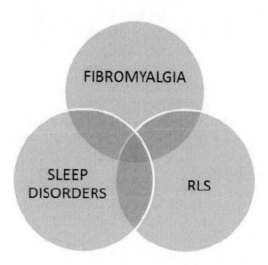

Figure 1. Overlap between RLS, fibromyalgia and other sleep disorders.

Those entities orbit around and sometimes overlap in those patients. RLS is considered a sleep disorder but fibromyalgia patients have insomnia regardless of RLS symptoms. The slow wave invasion in other sleep cycles is by far the classical electroencephalic alteration in the sleep of fibromyalgia patients. But that does not bring any new connections to the intricate pathophysiology of this condition. RLS in itself might not have a physiopathology that justifies this overlapping with fibromyalgia. Conceptually, fibromyalgia patients have a decreased pain threshold in trigger points that makes the pain status more severe regarding the intensity, duration, triggering, frequency and other components of pain. There is not a resemblance to RLS basic physiopathology that has a restricted time schedule to surface, has different intensities in each patient, different frequencies and many other related comorbidities.

The only intervention that successfully improves the quality of life in all fibromyalgia patients is physiotherapy in several approaches. The importance of exercise in RLS has been discussed. So, we can conclude that physical exercise in general might be a successful intervention for those patients.

The patients afflicted by RLS or other sleep disorders could also benefit from a sleep hygiene program such as that described in a recent article by Orlandi et al. [38]. They analyzed an experimental group randomly chosen among patients of two different healthcare facilities in the city of São Paulo, Brazil. All the patients had had the same first evaluation using the Pittsburgh Sleep Quality Index, validated for the Portuguese language and the Fibromyalgia Impact Questionnaire (FIQ), specifically for assessing the impact of fibromyalgia on the patient´s functional capacity, and also validated for Brazil. All patients received a booklet containing information about the disease, but only the control group received sleep hygiene instructions. Besides the sleep hygiene discussed in the respective chapter in this book, they also advised the patients to dress warmly at night to avoid contractures. All sleep hygiene points were read and explained to each patient of the experimental group, emphasizing the daily application of those instructions aided by a sleep diary, in which the patients should describe, in the last 15 days of treatment, their nights of sleep and the hours preceding bedtime. After three months, the patients returned to the clinic to be reassessed (second meeting). During those three months, patients and authors had no contact.

The final result was obtained from 70 women. The mean age of the patients in the control group was 55.2 ± 7.12 years, and in the experimental group, 53.5 ± 8.89 years (P = 0.392). They analyzed the sleep diaries in objective questions:

I.   More than 30 minutes to fall asleep
II.   Sleep again with difficulty
III.   Sleep again easily
IV.   Alcohol intake
V.   Inadequate food at night
VI.   Physical activity
VII.   Took medicines (sleeping pills)
VIII. Non-repairing sleep
IX.   Range of fatigue (0 to 4) during the day
X.   Range of fatigue (0 to 4) during the evening
XI.   Mean bedtime
XII.   Mean waking up time

Only variable III showed statistical differences between the groups. That question regards the number of days the patient woke up during the night and had no difficulty falling asleep again: while the control group had difficulty falling sleep again on 5.71±6.19 days, the experimental group had this difficulty on 2.91±4.35 days (p=0.031). If both groups went to bed and woke up at the same time the experimental group had an increased sleep efficiency on average. In the experimental group reductions in the following measures were observed: pain Visual Analogue Scale (VAS) (P = 0.028); fatigue (P = 0.021); and PSQI component 1 (P = 0.030), which relates to the subjective quality of sleep.

So, to conclude, the results of this study have shown an improvement in the subjective sleep quality and in the results of the VAS pain in patients with FM receiving sleep hygiene instructions. It is an important result for all physiotherapists working in the field. The protocol can be applied to RLS patients adding up the sleep hygiene points directed specifically for RLS patients also discussed in this book in the sleep hygiene chapter.

While TENS for RLS was not tested in large populations, TENS in fibromyalgia is associated with improvements such as a decrease in pain levels in addition to physiotherapy exercises. Carbonario et al. 2014 [39] used high intensity TENS adjunctive to physiotherapy including aerobic exercise and muscular chain stretching.

In their discussion, they comment that high intensity and low frequency TENS is usually applied in acute pain cases. They also report that this approach did not improve sleep patterns in those patients; actually, the control group that had physiotherapy only showed an improvement in sleep patterns. Another group studied TENS allied to physiotherapy, showing good results in the short term, also with a pain decrease [40]. They suggest that this might be important for daily treatment in physiotherapy. The important concept is that TENS might help in both fibromyalgia and RLS, probably with different frequencies and intensities.

Hamilton et al. evaluated a model that places sleep disorder as a predictor of fibromyalgia [20]. They argue that pain would be the mediator of the relationship between the disturbed sleep and physical disability. Indeed, from the more practical point of view, physiotherapy is used in order to cope with fibromyalgia, but the symptoms do fluctuate over the years, as stated in the article discussion, not followed by any biological markers that justified those changes. This is the reason that pushed me to show the relationship between those disorders in a Venn diagram.

From my point of view they are orbiting around the patient like our planet orbits around the sun. They might have attraction forces between them that change the final outcome by adding up forces upon the patient. So health professionals must see each one of these disorders and the final vector force that strikes the patient. On each patient one of the disorders will appear the strongest, and therefore this disorder should be attacked first.

Fibromyalgia, just like RLS, has not been understood in its physiopathology and it is known that pain medicines usually used to treat other conditions do not work in fibromyalgia patients, as they refer in daily practice. In western culture, when a disorder is not fully understood it is considered mysterious, untreatable. My concept is far removed from this point of view; if the patient has to stop and stretch two or three times a day and exercise once a day to bear the symptoms of this painful syndrome it is a successful and secure treatment. In terms of working hours and social security affairs, this might or not be a problem for the patient in terms of disability, depending on the type of work and each country's laws.

It does seem reasonable that those kinds of patients do not work night shifts, as we would recommend for idiopathic RLS patients. The fact that we do live in an increasingly sedentary and sleep-deprived society does not help those patients to blend in with the regular working force. The important consideration is that a successful treatment or intervention does allow the patient to continue to have a productive life in an adapted way. In daily practice, as the readers start to ask their patients about their sleeping habits, they will face a great challenge, maybe even worse than convincing patients to stretch and exercise frequently. The fact that good sleep hygiene demands time is the greater challenge imposed on all health professionals. In this sense maybe educating the fibromyalgia patient is the decisive conduct one must undertake to successfully attract the patient to this intervention.

The physiotherapist has an interesting position in a multidisciplinary team dealing with fibromyalgia patients. In my research when preparing to write this chapter, massage therapy was separate from physiotherapy.

That mistake is repeated in many reviews and it seems that massage therapy of any kind would be considered an alternative medicine that doctors would not usually recommend. For the non-physiotherapist readers of this book, I would like to clarify that massage therapy is a resource that physiotherapists study and apply, just like electrotherapy or thermotherapy, and it can be a regular part of a physiotherapy section. Massage therapy also has an obvious strong and relieving effect on fibromyalgia patients, regardless of whether they have RLS or any other sleep disorder.

References

[1] Pigeon WR, Yurcheshen M. Behavioral Sleep Medicine Interventions for Restless Legs Syndrome and Periodic Limb Movement Disorder. *Sleep medicine clinics.* 2009;4(4):487-94.

[2] Desseilles M, Dang-Vu T, Schabus M, Sterpenich V, Maquet P, Schwartz S. Neuroimaging insights into the pathophysiology of sleep disorders. *Sleep.* 2008;31(6):777-94.

[3] Ohayon MM, O'Hara R, Vitiello MV. Epidemiology of restless legs syndrome: a synthesis of the literature. *Sleep medicine reviews.* 16(4):283-95.

[4] Lin CH, Wu VC, Li WY, Sy HN, Wu SL, Chang CC, et al. Restless legs syndrome in end-stage renal disease: a multicenter study in Taiwan. *European journal of neurology: the official journal of the European Federation of Neurological Societies.* 2013;20(7):1025-31.

[5] Cho YW, Na GY, Lim JG, Kim SH, Kim HS, Earley CJ, et al. Prevalence and clinical characteristics of restless legs syndrome in diabetic peripheral neuropathy: comparison with chronic osteoarthritis. *Sleep medicine.* 2013;14(12):1387-92.

[6]   Stehlik R, Arvidsson L, Ulfberg J. Restless legs syndrome is common among female patients with fibromyalgia. *European neurology.* 2009;61(2):107-11.

[7]   Buchfuhrer MJ. Strategies for the treatment of restless legs syndrome. Neurotherapeutics: the journal of the American Society for Experimental *NeuroTherapeutics.* 2012;9(4):776-90.

[8]   Medicine AAoS. *International classification of sleep disorders, revised: diagnostic and coding manual.* 3rd ed. Chicago, Illinois: American Academy of Sleep Medicine; 2001. 208 p.

[9]   Dickel MJ, Renfrow SD, Moore PT, Berry RB. Rapid eye movement sleep periodic leg movements in patients with spinal cord injury. *Sleep.* 1994;17(8):733-8.

[10] Salminen AV, Manconi M, Rimpila V, Luoto TM, Koskinen E, Ferri R, et al. Disconnection between periodic leg movements and cortical arousals in spinal cord injury. *Journal of clinical sleep medicine: JCSM : official publication of the American Academy of Sleep Medicine.* 2013;9(11):1207-9.

[11] Brown TG. On the nature of the fundamental activity of the nervous centres; together with an analysis of the conditioning of rhythmic activity in progression, and a theory of the evolution of function in the nervous system. *J Physiol.* 1914;48(1):18-46.

[12] Barriere G, Cazalets JR, Bioulac B, Tison F, Ghorayeb I. The restless legs syndrome. *Prog Neurobiol.* 2005;77(3):139-65.

[13] Mello MC, Natal CL, Cunha JM, Tufik S. Epidemiologia do padrão de sono em adultos desportistas portadores de lesão medular. *Revista portuguesa de medicina desportiva.* 1995;13:89-100.

[14] Allen RP, Barker PB, Wehrl F, Song HK, Earley CJ. MRI measurement of brain iron in patients with restless legs syndrome. *Neurology.* 2001;56(2):263-5.

[15] Littner MR, Kushida C, Anderson WM, Bailey D, Berry RB, Hirshkowitz M, et al. Practice parameters for the dopaminergic treatment of restless legs syndrome and periodic limb movement disorder. *Sleep.* 2004;27(3):557-9.

[16] Vignatelli L, Billiard M, Clarenbach P, Garcia-Borreguero D, Kaynak D, Liesiene V, et al. EFNS guidelines on management of restless legs syndrome and periodic limb movement disorder in sleep. *European journal of neurology: the official journal of the European Federation of Neurological Societies.* 2006;13(10):1049-65.

[17] Paulus W, Schomburg ED. Dopamine and the spinal cord in restless legs syndrome: does spinal cord physiology reveal a basis for augmentation? *Sleep medicine reviews.* 2006;10(3):185-96.

[18] Esteves AM, de Mello MT, Pradella-Hallinan M, Tufik S. Effect of acute and chronic physical exercise on patients with periodic leg movements. *Medicine and science in sports and exercise.* 2009;41(1):237-42.

[19] Staedt J, Wassmuth F, Ziemann U, Hajak G, Ruther E, Stoppe G. Pergolide: treatment of choice in restless legs syndrome (RLS) and nocturnal myoclonus syndrome (NMS). A double-blind randomized crossover trial of pergolide versus L-Dopa. *Journal of neural transmission* (Vienna, Austria: 1996). 1997;104(4-5):461-8.

[20] Hamilton NA, Pressman M, Lillis T, Atchley R, Karlson C, Stevens N. Evaluating Evidence for the Role of Sleep in Fibromyalgia: A Test of the Sleep and Pain Diathesis Model. *Cognitive therapy and research.* 2012;36(6):806-14.

[21] Trenkwalder C, Benes H, Grote L, Happe S, Hogl B, Mathis J, et al. Cabergoline compared to levodopa in the treatment of patients with severe restless legs syndrome: results from a multi-center, randomized, active controlled trial. Movement disorders: *official journal of the Movement Disorder Society.* 2007;22(5):696-703.

[22] Bogan RK. Ropinirole treatment for restless legs syndrome. *Expert opinion on pharmacotherapy.* 2008;9(4):611-23.

[23] Hening WA, Allen RP, Ondo WG, Walters AS, Winkelman JW, Becker P, et al. Rotigotine improves restless legs syndrome: a 6-month randomized, double-blind, placebo-controlled trial in the United States. Movement disorders: *official journal of the Movement Disorder Society.* 2010;25(11):1675-83.

[24] Partinen M, Hirvonen K, Jama L, Alakuijala A, Hublin C, Tamminen I, et al. Open-label study of the long-term efficacy and safety of pramipexole in patients with Restless Legs Syndrome (extension of the PRELUDE study). *Sleep medicine.* 2008;9(5):537-41.

[25] Turjanski N, Lees AJ, Brooks DJ. Striatal dopaminergic function in restless legs syndrome: 18F-dopa and 11C-raclopride PET studies. *Neurology.* 1999;52(5):932-7.

[26] Earley CJ, Kuwabara H, Wong DF, Gamaldo C, Salas RE, Brasic JR, et al. Increased synaptic dopamine in the putamen in restless legs syndrome. *Sleep.* 2013;36(1):51-7.

[27] Cho YW, Allen RP, Earley CJ. Lower molecular weight intravenous iron dextran for restless legs syndrome. *Sleep medicine*. 2013;14(3): 274-7.

[28] Trenkwalder C, Benes H, Grote L, Garcia-Borreguero D, Hogl B, Hopp M, et al. Prolonged release oxycodone-naloxone for treatment of severe restless legs syndrome after failure of previous treatment: a double-blind, randomised, placebo-controlled trial with an open-label extension. *Lancet neurology*. 2013;12(12):1141-50.

[29] Clemens S, Rye D, Hochman S. Restless legs syndrome Revisiting the dopamine hypothesis from the spinal cord perspective. *Neurology*. 2006;67(1):125-30.

[30] Nilsson S, Levi R, Nordstrom A. Treatment-resistant sensory motor symptoms in persons with SCI may be signs of restless legs syndrome. *Spinal cord*. 2011;49(6):754-6.

[31] Irkec C, Vuralli D, Karacay Ozkalayci S. Restless legs syndrome as the initial presentation of multiple sclerosis. *Case reports in medicine*. 2013;2013:290719.

[32] Lee MS, Choi YC, Lee SH, Lee SB. Sleep-related periodic leg movements associated with spinal cord lesions. *Movement disorders: official journal of the Movement Disorder Society*. 1996;11(6):719-22.

[33] De Mello MT, Esteves AM, Tufik S. Comparison between dopaminergic agents and physical exercise as treatment for periodic limb movements in patients with spinal cord injury. *Spinal cord*. 2004;42(4):218-21.

[34] Mitchell UH. Nondrug-related aspect of treating Ekbom disease, formerly known as restless legs syndrome. *Neuropsychiatric disease and treatment*. 2011;7:251-7.

[35] Davis JC, Bryan S, Marra CA, Sharma D, Chan A, Beattie BL, et al. An economic evaluation of resistance training and aerobic training versus balance and toning exercises in older adults with mild cognitive impairment. *PloS one*. 2013;8(5):e63031.

[36] Giummarra MJ, Bradshaw JL. The phantom of the night: restless legs syndrome in amputees. *Medical hypotheses*. 2010;74(6):968-72.

[37] Skidmore FM, Drago V, Foster PS, Heilman KM. Bilateral restless legs affecting a phantom limb, treated with dopamine agonists. *Journal of neurology, neurosurgery, and psychiatry*. 2009;80(5):569-70.

[38] Orlandi AC, Ventura C, Gallinaro AL, Costa RA, Lage LV. Melhora da dor, do cansaço e da qualidade subjetiva do sono por meio de orientações de higiene do sono em pacientes com fibromialgia. *Revista Brasileira de Reumatologia*. 2012;52:672-8.

[39] Carbonario F, Matsutani LA, Yuan SL, Marques AP. Effectiveness of high-frequency transcutaneous electrical nerve stimulation at tender points as adjuvant therapy for patients with fibromyalgia. *European journal of physical and rehabilitation medicine*. 2013;49(2):197-204.

[40] Mutlu B, Paker N, Bugdayci D, Tekdos D, Kesiktas N. Efficacy of supervised exercise combined with transcutaneous electrical nerve stimulation in women with fibromyalgia: a prospective controlled study. *Rheumatology international*. 2013;33(3):649-55.

Chapter 5

Habits that Might Trigger RLS and PLM

Abstract

In this chapter the reader will learn that there are habits that might trigger RLS episodes. The reader will learn the concepts of sleep hygiene and there will be a discussion about the application of those concepts in the daily life of physiotherapy patients using a sleep diary. Scientific evidence discussing the methodology and outcomes of the application of those concepts will also be shown.

RLS, PLM and its Triggers

The most severe cases of RLS are followed by innumerous interventions the patients come up with. Sometimes those measures are not helpful, and sometimes they might worsen the symptoms.

In my preparatory research for this book, I have searched for many alternative therapies that might benefit RLS patients. I have found websites, nonscientific news, blogs, and books which are sold in American online bookstores. The impressive amount of information made it impossible to cover it all. But vitamins or diets were the most present. There is no scientific evidence to support any of those measures.

The scientific evidence supports sleep hygiene habits. Sleep deprivation is largely connected to worsening RLS episodes.

PLM is not really linked to sleep hygiene habits in the literature; on the other hand, as was discussed before, it does have a response in the number of events occurring after exercise. If one should consider exercise and practice inserting it in sleep hygiene concepts, avoiding exercise after the evening, then it can be considered that PLM does have a response to sleep hygiene concepts.

Concept of Sleep Hygiene

The concept of sleep hygiene can be applied to all kinds of patients. According to Gigli et al., [1] this concept was developed in 1977 by Peter Hauri, containing a set of sleep-promoting rules, considered the fundament for sleep hygiene techniques. Indeed, sleep habits have been considered important to good health and "inadequate sleep hygiene" was included as a sleep disorder in the International Classification of Sleep Disorders. The article discusses how this concept has already been written about by Paolo Mantegazza, a scientist and professor in the Medical School of the University of Pavia, Italy. This article shows citations of the original book published by Mantegazza in 1864 dealing with sleep hygiene [1]. The important point is that, for RLS patients, sleep hygiene measures are essential and must be strictly followed.

Sleep hygiene is the expression used to define sleep habits that resemble our physiology according to our age. When we are newborn babies those measures are usually followed so that the baby can also feed and grow up accordingly. But when we reach adult life we have completely disrupted good sleeping habits and turn out to have sleep disorders.

Those habits are so completely forgotten or have not been completely developed that adults in the regular population might have no idea at all that bad sleeping habits might bring about chronic conditions such as obesity, diabetes and others. People in general take a long time to link bad work performance and lapses in memory to not getting enough sleep. Usually people link diurnal somnolence to bad sleep and they go to the doctor only for that reason.

Before inserting good sleep habits in daily life, the health professional must explain why this is so important. The intervention program must have deadlines. The average number of hours slept can be measured easily with actigraphy for 1 or 2 weeks in cases where the sleeping pattern is completely fragmented [2].

Advice for good sleeping habits:

- Avoid taking long naps during the day; it can cause insomnia. If daytime sleepiness becomes overwhelming, limit yourself to a single nap of 30 minutes or less, preferably after lunch. Avoid stimulants such as caffeine, nicotine, and alcohol too close to bedtime.
- Exercise can promote good sleep. Vigorous exercise should be taken in the morning or late afternoon.
- Avoid large meals just before bedtime. If you have a condition such as gastro esophageal reflux disease, which may cause coughing or choking, avoid eating within 3 hours of bedtime.
- Do not go to bed hungry. Have a light snack one hour or several hours before bedtime if necessary.
- Ensure adequate exposure to natural light. This is particularly important for older people who may not venture outside as frequently as children and adults. Light exposure helps maintain a healthy sleep-wake cycle.
- Establish a regular relaxing bedtime routine such as taking a hot bath, or listening to relaxing music.
- Try to avoid emotionally upsetting conversations and activities before trying to go to sleep. Avoid violent and noisy programs on T.V.
- If you like watching TV in the bedroom, set the timer to 20 minutes. The light emitted by the TV or the laptop is enough to trigger the wakefulness system in your body.
- Don't bring your problems to bed. Write them down in a notebook and go to sleep.
- To keep your bed healthy, change your pillow once a year. Watch out for the right size of the pillow: it should be as high as the distance between your shoulder and your neck. The best position to sleep is on your side.
- Be vigilant in cleaning the room. Keep the walls free from mold.
- Associate your bed with sleep. It's not a good idea to use your bed to watch TV, listen to the radio, or read.
- Make sure that the sleep environment is pleasant and relaxing. The bed should be comfortable.
- The room should not be too hot or cold, or too bright.

- Keep a regular sleep schedule of 7-8 hours of sleep. Go to bed and wake up at the same time every day, even on weekends. This will help the development of a consistent sleep-wake rhythm.
- Make sure you are pleasantly tired before going to bed.
- Do not stay in bed for more than 20-30 minutes if experiencing insomnia. In this case, get up and do something boring and repetitive such as reading an uninteresting book.
- Use a sleep diary to help integrate those measures in your daily life.

Table 4. Sleep diary

SLEEP DIARY							
DAY	MONDAY	TUESDAY	WEDNESDAY	THURSDAY	FRIDAY	SATURDAY	SUNDAY
TIME THAT I WENT TO BED							
TIME THAT I FELL ASLEEP							
WOKE UP DURING THE NIGHT (NUMBER OF TIMES)							
WAKING UP TIME							
NAPS DURING THE DAY							
RLS SYMPTOMS STARTED							
RLS SYMPTOMS ENDED							
SLEEP RATING (VERY BAD, BAD, STANDARD, GOOD OR GREAT							

Scientific Evidence

Orlandi et al. analyzed the effectiveness of sleep hygiene measures in 70 women afflicted by fibromyalgia. Both groups received information about the disease and a sleep diary, but only the experimental group received sleep hygiene tips. The authors used the Fibromyalgia Impact Questionnaire and The Pittsburgh Sleep Quality Index make comparisons before and after the three-month intervention. The experimental group showed a decrease in pain and fatigue, and a significant reduction in falling asleep after waking up in the middle of the night [3].

Custers and Van den Bulck [4] evaluated whether the availability of the Internet and TV in the bedroom and overall Internet use and TV viewing were related to sleep variables such as circadian disturbances, total sleep time and fatigue. They analyzed a sample of 711 residents of Flanders, Belgium, and found some evidence of time shifting: Internet access in the bedroom predicted a later bedtime ($\beta = .12$, $p < .05$) and later rising time ($\beta = .11$, $p < .05$) on weekdays and later bedtime ($\beta = .10$, $p < .001$) on weekends.

Internet use volume predicted a later bedtime ($\beta = .10$, $p < .001$) and rising time ($\beta = .07$, $p < .05$) on weekends, and TV viewing predicted later bedtime ($\beta = .10$, $p < .05$) on weekends. However, neither the availability of the Internet or TV in the bedroom, nor the volume of Internet use or TV viewing was a significant predictor of reduced total sleep time or fatigue. This study clarifies that those measures might not be too harsh depending on the case and patients do not have to take the TV out of their rooms. In daily practice, many patients report that they like to listen to the TV to get to sleep.

Another study tried to clarify the myth of caffeine effects, the most used stimulant present in many beverages. This study compared the potential disruptive effects on sleep of a fixed dose of caffeine (400 mg) administered at 0, 3, and 6 hours prior to habitual bedtime relative to a placebo on self-reported sleep in the home.

Results demonstrated a moderate dose of caffeine at bedtime, 3 hours prior to bedtime, or 6 hours prior to bedtime each have significant effects on sleep disturbance relative to the placebo ($p < 0.05$ for all). Their conclusion is that caffeine does disrupt sleep and the better sleep hygiene measure is to avoid caffeine before bedtime [5].

Conclusion

Sleep hygiene is a valuable concept and a sleep diary is an excellent tool to manage sleep disorders. In RLS it is essential for a more effective outcome as sleep deprivation clearly worsens the RLS symptoms. It is important to keep in mind that this is a part of the treatment.

References

[1]   Gigli GL, Valente M. Should the definition of "sleep hygiene" be antedated of a century? A historical note based on an old book by Paolo Mantegazza, rediscovered. To place in a new historical context the development of the concept of sleep hygiene. *Neurological sciences: official journal of the Italian Neurological Society and of the Italian Society of Clinical Neurophysiology.* 2013;34(5):755-60.

[2]   Telles S, Corrêa E, Caversan B, Mattos J, Alves R. *The Actigraph Clinical Significance. Endereço para correspondência: Susana CL Telles Av Dr Arnaldo.*455:2o.

[3]   Orlandi AC, Ventura C, Gallinaro AL, Costa RA, Lage LV. Melhora da dor, do cansaço e da qualidade subjetiva do sono por meio de orientações de higiene do sono em pacientes com fibromialgia. *Revista Brasileira de Reumatologia.* 2012;52:672-8.

[4]   Custers K, Van den Bulck J. Television viewing, internet use, and self-reported bedtime and rise time in adults: implications for sleep hygiene recommendations from an exploratory cross-sectional study. *Behavioral sleep medicine.* 2012;10(2):96-105.

[5]   Drake C, Roehrs T, Shambroom J, Roth T. Caffeine effects on sleep taken 0, 3, or 6 hours before going to bed. *Journal of clinical sleep medicine: JCSM: official publication of the American Academy of Sleep Medicine.* 2013;9(11):1195-200.

Chapter 6

New Physical
Therapy Approaches

Abstract

In this chapter the reader will learn about new physical therapy evaluation procedures and approaches being studied in peer review papers by health professionals from all over the world. All the steps of the evaluation are exposed in tables, texts, charts and figures to make it easier for the reader, as the evaluation is essential for choosing the right intervention protocol. Those are new approaches and each one must be further studied by all readers before their application in daily practice such as treadmill, bicycles, lumbar support belt, near infrared light. The chapter finishes in an overview of pain concepts and a discussion of possible physiological mechanisms for each intervention discussed in the chapter.

Introduction

Patients afflicted by RLS and PLM can be treated with several medicines. Some of those medicines have serious side effects and patients might not stand this kind of treatment. Regardless of the clinical trials and their indications, patients might have a better handling of RLS if approached by physical therapy by a specialized health professional. Each country has its own legislation about the health professional responsible for applying those approaches.

Physical therapy is usually studied as one block intervention as if there was only one resource or protocol. This is a problem detected also in a systematic review [1].

The reader should be alerted that when a systematic review shows a low level of evidence it might be related to the kind of methodological approach used in the studies available in the literature. The area of physical therapy must be examined in more detail, comparing its own results evaluated by its own tools, whether they are functional outcomes, quality of life questionnaires or statistical analysis. For the current time case studies might also be quite valuable for our area.

Daily Practice:
The pt. Evaluation and Procedures

The physiotherapeutic consultation must have a specific anamnesis for sleep disturbances with the use of Epworth´s Sleepiness Scale [2] and the Pittsburg Questionnaire on Quality of Sleep [3]:

In Table 4 the possible related disorders that are presented in our physiotherapists clinics are shown. Other conditions such as kidney disease, pregnancy, and anemia might be related to but they are not the subject of this book.

The reader can choose to apply scales to address the severity of RLS, sleep quality and diurnal somnolence. The clinical investigation, though, does not use those scales.

Following those tables there are the questions, comments and interventions shown in Table 13, organized to show that the pt. must address questions related to other modalities of sleep disturbance.

The importance of sleep hygiene has already been discussed in Chapter 5. In this chapter we will discuss the call to action for methodology in our intervention program.

Sleep deprivation is a hidden epidemic in our times. It seems that in many countries it is considered natural to sleep only 5 or 6 hours a night. Many studies' have already been reported regarding the risks of sleep deprivation. In this chapter we will also discuss an intervention program in this area.

Sleep ergonomics must be taken seriously by physiotherapists. It is clear that if your patient assumes the wrong position for 6 hours a day, this will be the ideal environment for chronic musculoskeletal pain and bad posture. This will lead to a poor sleep quality and even to sleep avoidance if the pain escalates in severity. The physiotherapist might come up with new evaluation questions. The following tables show the evaluation protocol for each item in this book:

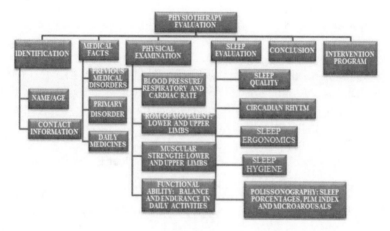

Figure 2. Fluxogram showing steps in physiotherapy evaluation.

The circadian rhythm is a topic that would fill an entire book. In this chapter we will discuss a small fraction of this topic to put into action. RLS patients tend to sleep later because of their symptoms. We must have the clear objective of making the patient sleep earlier, in addition to the results of the main intervention.

Diurnal somnolence is one of the major sleep disturbances patients will report. When it is present, it is usually linked to a more severe RLS and/or PLM. It might decrease productivity in work, it might affect one's social life, and it might trigger other health problems. It must be one of our main objectives in treating the RLS patient.

Insomnia is a separate sleep disorder that can be related to RLS or can be related to an acute or chronic episode. In this case sending the patient to a medical doctor or psychologist is absolutely essential. Our intervention might focus on relaxing techniques and even biofeedback to stress management. If the patient is not treated for insomnia, he will not see any improvement in diurnal somnolence and connected symptoms.

Table 4. Section 2 of pt. evaluation: Medical Facts

Previous medical disorder	Spinal cord injury, limb amputation, stroke, metabolic syndrome, fibromyalgia, neuromuscular disorders, cardiac disorders
Primary disorder	PLM during sleep and or RLS – apply International Restless Legs Syndrome Study Group[4] evaluation in this case
Daily medicines	Frequency and dosage: attention for drugs that affect sleep

The physiotherapist, who especially works in amputee rehabilitation, must be alert to the possibility of RLS in the amputated lower limb. In a 2009 article, evaluating 283 amputees due to a peripheral vascular disease or trauma, Giummarra and Bradsham detected 13% afflicted by RLS [5]. There is no consensus of physiotherapeutic approach to amputees afflicted by RLS. It is a recent discovery, but the authors suggested that it must have a different approach from that of phantom pain.

Table 5. Section 3 of pt. evaluation: Physical Examination

Blood pressure, respiratory and cardiac rate	All in rest position, after entrance in the room and sitting quietly in a chair
ROM of movement	Review the subject if necessary [6]
Muscle testing	Review the subject if necessary [7]
Functional ability	In general idiopathic RLS/PLM patients have no motor disabilities. Those might come from adjunctive conditions our patients have

Table 6. Section 4 of pt. evaluation: Sleep evaluation

Epworth sleepiness scale	Very useful to detect diurnal somnolence
Pittsburg questionnaire	Very useful to detect sleep habits
Polysomnography: sleep percentages, PLM index and microarousals	Important to give an idea of the severity of PLM or other sleep disorders such as sleep apnea

How to apply Epworth Sleepiness Scale: This scale is self-administered. It must be explained that the patient will be asked to rate from 0-3 the chance of dozing off during certain day-to-day situations [2]. There are eight situations that are added together and can total from 0 to 24. A score greater than 10 is considered excessive diurnal somnolence.

How to apply the Pittsburg questionnaire: The Pittsburg Sleep Quality Index is a self-rated questionnaire which aims to assess sleep quality and disturbances over the last month. Nineteen individual items generate seven "component" scores: subjective sleep quality, sleep latency, sleep duration, habitual sleep efficiency, sleep disturbances, use of sleeping medication, and daytime dysfunction. A sum of scores>5 means that the patient is a poor sleeper [3].

How to apply International Restless Legs Syndrome Scale: This is a self-applied 10-question questionnaire in that the patient must rate the RLS symptoms choosing from 4 items on each question. The score classifies the severity of RLS: NONE (ZERO Points, 1-10 (mild), moderate (11-20), severe (21-30), very severe (31-40).

Polysomnography

The study test is a great opportunity to assess the severity of the sleep disorder, although it is not the physiotherapist's role to understand this test in detail.

Conclusion

One needs to assess and gather information previously reported to sustain a decisive conclusion and effective intervention. Physical examination is crucial whenever there are previous disabilities. Sleep evaluation is based on a standard diurnal somnolence scale and a questionnaire that indicates sleep hygiene habits.

Objectives

- Guide, favor and readapt the client/patient to the program of aerobic exercises.

- Determine the performance conditions for the aerobic program and, if necessary, recondition the client/patient through specific kinesiotherapy adequate for each case in order to prepare the patient for the aerobic program, establishing compensatory pauses and reassess the strategies for physiotherapeutic intervention.

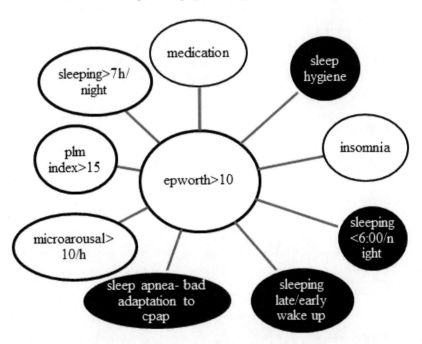

Figure 3. The painted spheres are situations in which the physiotherapist might help. The white spheres are situations in which the medical doctor might help. All of them are connected to Epworth>10 and excessive diurnal somnolence.

Intervention

a. Treadmill and Bicycles

The key point about PLM and RLS is that they improve immediately after movement. This theme has already been discussed in the physiopathology chapter. The scientific basis for exercise decreasing PLM has not been completely unraveled. But PLM has already been approached by programs including aerobic exercises (treadmill bicycles or treadmill) varying in intensity, duration, number of sessions and follow-up, with good results.

Lower limb strengthening exercises have also been applied along with aerobics, demonstrating good results [8, 9]. The chronic character of these disorders reflects what happens in practice: the results are maintained only when the patient is adherent to the program.

There is evidence that physical exercise decreases the symptoms of PLM; however, there is still no consensus about it [9]. No type of exercise has been defined as effective; however, the majority of protocols include treadmill bicycles and other exercises that vary according to the protocol. The physiotherapist who works in spinal cord injury rehabilitation must be alert because the patients can manifest PLM [10]. There is evidence of an improvement in the symptoms of these patients in protocols involving adapted treadmill bicycles.

b. Lumbar Support Belt and Periodic Leg Movements

A lumbar corset is traditionally applied for lower back pain symptoms caused by innumerous vertebral column affections originating from temporary musculoskeletal disorders or from more serious orthopedic disorders. Of course, each disorder has a different outcome with the lumbar support treatment. Recently, Yee et al. [11] reported a randomized trial to evaluate the effect of a postoperative corset on the outcome of lumbar arthrodesis for 8 weeks in patients afflicted with a degenerative spinal condition. The authors compared physical examination, radiographs, and functional outcome questionnaires (the Dallas Pain Questionnaire (DPQ) and the Short Form-36 (SF-36) preoperatively and at one year and two years following the surgery for 37 patients in contrast with 35 patients who did not use lumbar support. This was a long-period evaluation one and two years after the surgery. This study does not indicate a significant advantage or disadvantage for the use of a postoperative lumbar corset following spinal arthrodesis for degenerative conditions of the lumbar spine. It was classified as Therapeutic Level I for the level of evidence.

In a systematic review of spinal stenosis[1] there is a comparison of regular lumbar corsets and devices that take away the patient's weight through a lifting technique in treadmill walking. In this case there is no significant difference in the final outcome.

The corsets can be used in osteoporosis cases. In the market they range from traditional corsets to very highly technological corsets designed to guarantee more freedom of movement to the patient. Talic et al. [12] compared plaster corsets with ortosis for treating osteoporotic fractures in the thoracolumbar spine. A plaster corset gives stability; patients with orthoses are more mobile without skin changes. Orthosis is recommended for most disciplined patients and the best treatment is that all the patients have a plaster corset for six weeks, followed by three-point orthoses until recovery.

The Case Discussion

Ishizu et al. [13] reported a 77-year-old woman with Restless Legs Syndrome [13] and periodic limb movement (PLM). This patient had already been treated with clonazepam (2.5 mg/day) and valproate (400 mg/day) at 77 years of age, and the symptoms clearly ameliorated but were closely followed by trunk ataxia and nystagmus. Without the drugs she was cleared of the side effects but RLS symptoms turned back. A cervical MRI revealed focal compression of the spinal cord by osteophytes at C5-C6 (more severe on the left side). Motor evoked potentials with transcranial magnetic stimulation revealed a mild delay in the central conduction time.

The treatment was then followed by the use of a lumbar corset. Consequently, the PLM symptoms during sleep and RLS symptoms disappeared.

To discuss why this device has worked we must analyze the biomechanics of the alignment of our lumbar vertebrae. Those five vertebrae are the largest and most weight-bearing vertebrae of our body. They are covered and surrounded by muscle, nerves, blood vessels and visceral structure vital to our survival. We will adapt our posture to protect vital structures and this might end up in a nerve compression or herniation. Solomonow et al. [14] reported on the neuromuscular changes leading to increased instability in the lumbar column caused by repetitive flexion extension movements with or without load. The changes in terms of instability in a chronic fashion are very important for our evaluation.

The CPG is probably located in the lumbar spinal cord in humans. This is quite a challenging point: since its location is in a region so prone to neuromuscular stress, could inflammation molecules in charge and weight bearing/mobile function really endanger our CPG?

And could that turn into PLM and RLS, not only in spinal cord injury patients, but in all humans who are working or practicing sports that require repetitive flexion-extension movements?

a. Near Infrared Light and Restless Legs Syndrome

Another attempt at a non-drug treatment was undertaken to evaluate the efficacy of monochromatic infrared light in decreasing RLS symptoms. In a randomized study, the International Restless Legs Syndrome Study Group [15,16] evaluations were performed before, during and after applications. Thirty-four patients were submitted to 12 applications on the legs for 30 minutes. The results showed a continuous decrease in the symptoms of the treatment group when compared with the control group (P<0.001). The improvement was maintained for 4 weeks after the treatment, when compared to the basal results; however, there was a small trend of increasing symptoms after five weeks. The system used in this therapy was the Anodyne® with a wavelength of 890 nm, whose effect, theoretically, occurs due to the release of nitric acid and, consequently, a chain of biochemical reactions on the blood vessels which leads to a better local circulation. The same group compared two infrared wavelengths and frequencies. In this randomized experiment, 25 individuals were submitted to the same scheme of sessions of the previous study and were evaluated in the same fashion. The differences between the Anodyne® system and the one known as Heat Light® are the use of an infrared light of 650 nm in Heat Light®, and the frequencies of 292 Hz for the Anodyne® and 4698 Hz for the Heat Light®. Both equipment significantly improved the symptoms of RLS, with no significant difference between the two equipment [17]. No polysomnography or any sleep study was performed.

b. Transcutaneous Electrical Nervous Stimulation (TENS) and Restless Legs Syndrome

In terms of RLS intervention the are few scientific evidences. In a single revision of a non-drug treatment, the transcutaneous electrical neural stimulation (TENS) was used showing positive results [18]. In the clinical practice of idiopathic RLS, presenting a strong circadian mode of nocturnal appearance of the symptoms, the TENS would work if the patient applied it at home, after orientation from the physiotherapist.

Burbank et al. [19] were clearly inspired by the TENS to develop a vibrating pad. The developers were quite careful in developing an easy-to-use device, with proper "cool down" to lower the stimulus and a controller to manage the strength; they instructed the patients in a double-blind fashion. In the introduction of this chapter the comment that underlies all physiotherapy is that there can be no sham stimulus in our studies. What is more interesting is that in Part III the authors discuss how patients who believed they had been given the treatment pad scored lower in the IRRLS scale. Also, the physicians who evaluated the patients clinically found a better outcome in patients who had used the treatment vibrating pad, instead of the sound or light emission pad. It is quite likely that the patients who believed that the pad would work were able to hang on a more vigorous stimulus in amplitude; that is, for the neurophysiology of the nervous receptors and their impulse, reaching the level of nervous impulse of that modality.

The relationship between pain and Restless Legs Syndrome is largely reviewed by Winkelman et al. [20]. The interesting point made is that the RLS phenomenon can be viewed or classified as pain according to different perspectives of the phenomenon. For all pain classifications researchers usually try to link them to metaphors of the patients' daily life, and so the patients afflicted by RLS have many metaphors to explain those feelings.

Further developing this idea of the thresholds of RLS patients in the pt. daily practice means that the TENS amperage must be lower at the beginning of the treatment. But it should increase throughout the pt. sessions in order desensitize the patient, just like the pain cases we deal with in our daily practice.

Concepts of Pain - Theories

To better understand the vibrating pad and TENS the reader must understand the Neuronal Circuits that modulate pain.

Traditionally, the first theory proposed by Melzack and Wall in the 1960s: The *Gate Control Theory* that implies non-painful inputs close the gates to painful input, which prevents the pain sensation from travelling to the CNS. The site of this occurrence would be in the spinal cord level. This would happen anatomically in a pre-synaptic inhibition on dorsal root nociceptor fibers that synapse on nociceptors spinal neurons. The gate theory was the rationale for the idea behind the production and use of TENS, which is used quite often for complementary pain management. It brings partial results because the pain suppression is also modulated by the *Ascending and Descending Pain Suppression Mechanism* that climbs through ascending spinothalamic tracts.

Even though RSL is not pain, some patients do recognize it as pain, but it can be considered an uncomfortable sensation triggered in a lower amperage impulse, and that might have superior central nervous system modulation or it can be spinal cord phenomena only, as has already been addressed in this book.

This inside-out, uncomfortable feeling would have to come from or start in the lower back vertebrae, more specifically to transmit this impulse to the sciatic nerve, and follow to the tibialis nerve. In this level, the dopamine receptors located in the spinal cord would then perform accordingly, increasing this sensation. The movement or the vibration would then be the "gate" closing for this stimulus, causing a suppression of the uncomfortable feelings. When the counter-stimulus stops, it does not take long for the uncomfortable feelings to come back.

If it involves the superior nervous system, the modulation of pain by electrical brain stimulation results from the activation of descending inhibitory fibers, which modulate (block) the input and output of laminae I, II, V and VII neurons.

Conclusion

This text brings some start-up ideas for performing physiotherapy on RLS and PLM patients. Right now, as this is being written, someone might be making up a new approach. Physiotherapy has a lot to develop in terms of researches, approaches and most importantly, recognition of the efficacy of our approaches as a good form of treatment.

Sleep science is also very new. Its most famous disorder is sleep apnea which is handled by respiratory therapists through CPAP adaptation. It is becoming recognized as an important disease.

Patients will always search for the easiest way to handle their disorders. Just like using CPAP, all interventions described here are 15% pt. responsibility and 85% patient´s adherence. If the patient does not follow the exercise protocol, or does not turn on the TENS or vibrating pad every night, it will not convey proper handling of the RLS symptoms. Each patient will feel more stimulated with different approaches that can also be mixed and accumulate results. Those pt. approaches can also be alternated with the medicine approach.

There is always room for other pt. resources that might work, such as warm pads. Sometimes the simplest approach will be better for a patient who has already tried many different interventions.

Researches for the Future

As previously said, those approaches can be combined with other measures such as sleep hygiene, medication, and others.

TENS must be studied in detail, aiming at a comparison between the intensity of electrical stimulus, and the frequencies and shapes of waves according to modern equipment standards.

The different exercise approaches must be more developed and tested in larger populations. Many protocols can be developed.

The lumbar corset has already been studied but not for use in PLM patients such as in this case discussion.

It is quite possible that patients with secondary RLS due to hernia might benefit from a postural evaluation and intervention toward improving the hernia position and symptoms, which might also include surgical intervention.

The multidisciplinary team provides an outstanding opportunity for patients and professionals alike. The patient has increased chances of proper handling of RLS and PLM. The professionals have the opportunity of creating stronger and more convincing results that lead to better outcomes.

References

[1]   Macedo LG, Hum A, Kuleba L, Mo J, Truong L, Yeung M, et al. Physical therapy interventions for degenerative lumbar spinal stenosis: a systematic review. *Physical therapy.* 2013;93(12):1646-60.

[2]   Johns MW. A new method for measuring daytime sleepiness: the Epworth sleepiness scale. *Sleep.* 1991;14(6):540-5.

[3]   Buysse DJ, Reynolds CF, 3rd, Monk TH, Berman SR, Kupfer DJ. The Pittsburgh Sleep Quality Index: a new instrument for psychiatric practice and research. *Psychiatry research.* 1989;28(2):193-213.

[4]   Walters AS, LeBrocq C, Dhar A, Hening W, Rosen R, Allen RP, et al. Validation of the International Restless Legs Syndrome Study Group rating scale for restless legs syndrome. *Sleep medicine.* 2003;4(2):121-32.

[5]   Giummarra MJ, Bradshaw JL. The phantom of the night: restless legs syndrome in amputees. *Medical hypotheses.* 2009;74(6):968-72.

[6]   Norkin CC, White J. *Measurement of Joint Motion: A guide to Goniometry.* 4 ed. Philadelphia: F.A. Davis; 2009.

[7]   Kendall FP. Muscles: *Testing and Function with Posture and Pain:* Lippincott Williams & Wilkins; 2005.

[8]   Aurora RN, Chowdhuri S, Ramar K, Bista SR, Casey KR, Lamm CI, et al. The treatment of central sleep apnea syndromes in adults: practice parameters with an evidence-based literature review and meta-analyses. *Sleep.*35(1):17-40.

[9]   Pigeon WR, Yurcheshen M. Behavioral Sleep Medicine Interventions for Restless Legs Syndrome and Periodic Limb Movement Disorder. *Sleep medicine clinics.* 2009;4(4):487-94.

[10]   Telles SC, Alves RC, Chadi G. Periodic limb movements during sleep and restless legs syndrome in patients with ASIA A spinal cord injury. *J Neurol Sci.* 2011;303(1-2):119-23.

[11]   Yee AJ, Yoo JU, Marsolais EB, Carlson G, Poe-Kochert C, Bohlman HH, et al. Use of a postoperative lumbar corset after lumbar spinal arthrodesis for degenerative conditions of the spine. A prospective randomized trial. *The Journal of bone and joint surgery American volume.* 2008;90(10):2062-8.

[12]   Talic A, Kapetanovic J, Dizdar A. Effects of conservative treatment for osteoporotic thoracolumbal spine fractures. *Materia socio-medica.* 2012;24(1):16-20.

[13]   Ishizu T, Ohyagi Y, Furuya H, Araki T, Tobimatsu S, Yamada T, et al. [A patient with restless legs syndrome/periodic limb movement successfully treated by wearing a lumbar corset]. Rinsho shinkeigaku = *Clinical neurology.* 2001;41(7):438-41.

[14]   Solomonow M, Zhou BH, Lu Y, King KB. Acute repetitive lumbar syndrome: A multi-component insight into the disorder. *Journal of bodywork and movement therapies.* 2012;16(2):134-47.

[15]   Foundation RLS. RLS Medical Bulletin2005 4/7/2012. Available from: http://www.irlssg.org/

[16]   Mitchell UH. Use of near-infrared light to reduce symptoms associated with restless legs syndrome in a woman: a case report. *Journal of medical case reports.* 2010;4:286.

[17]   Mitchell UH, Myrer JW, Johnson AW, Hilton SC. Restless legs syndrome and near-infrared light: An alternative treatment option. *Physiotherapy theory and practice.* 2011;27(5):345-51.

[18]   Krueger BR. Restless legs syndrome and periodic movements of sleep. *Mayo Clinic proceedings.* 1990;65(7):999-1006.

[19]   Burbank F. Sleep improvement for restless legs syndrome patients. Part III: effect of treatment assignment belief on sleep improvement in

restless legs syndrome patients. A mediation analysis. *Journal of Parkinsonism and Restless Legs Syndrome.* 2013;3:23-9.

[20] Winkelman JW, Gagnon A, Clair AG. Sensory symptoms in restless legs syndrome: the enigma of pain. *Sleep medicine.* 2013;14(10):934-42.

Chapter 7

Actigraphy

Abstract

Actigraphy is a portable device composed by an accelerometer and memory for recording long time periods. It is useful to monitor PLM in the patient's natural environment, and it can be used to monitor the response of our intervention, sparing the patient another full night of polysomnography.

The data collected are displayed on a computer and the software analyzes the presence or absence of activity, and wake or sleep.

This chapter will discuss the use of actigraphy in PLM and RLS patients. The reader will learn about how to handle those devices and their softwares available on the market [1].

Introduction

As previously explained, the gold standard to diagnose sleep disorder is polysomnography in the case of PLM. RLS has a clinical diagnosis, as also explained in previous chapters. The scales to analyze the severity are available in the literature. But an actigraphy recording can be an objective device to track down the circadian disorder implied by RLS and PLM. The devices are approximately the size of a wrist watch and can be placed on the leg [1].

Digitalization

New models available on the market collect physical movement, sampling it several times per second and storing in 1-minute epochs. It is important to remember that those settings can be customized by the healthcare professionals. Some actigraphs record other parameters in addition to activity such as ambient light, skin temperature and sound. These additional features enhance the capabilities of actigraphs to record and provide data regarding circadian rhythms in the home environment.

Most actigraphs also have optional events buttons that the patient can push to mark events such as turning off lights and so on.

Internal Algorithms

There are three ways signals can be digitized:

1. Time above threshold: counts the amount of time per epoch that the motion signal is above a given threshold. However, neither the amplitude of the signal nor the acceleration of the movement are reflected in this strategy.
2. Zero crossing mode: counts the number of times per epoch that the signal crosses zero. However, neither the amplitude of the signal nor the acceleration of the movement are reflected in this strategy, and artifacts might be present.
3. Digital integration mode: samples the accelerometry output signals at a high rate and calculates the area under the curve for each epoch. This shows the amplitude and acceleration, but does not reflect the duration or frequency of the signal.

Computer Algorithms

Once the data are digitized, the information is downloaded to the software. Usually, computer algorithms are used to automatically score wake and sleep and to provide the user with summary statistics. Measures such as total sleep time, percentage of time spent asleep, total awake time, percentage of time spent awake, number of awakenings, time between awakenings and sleep onset latency are provided in the software.

Most commercial software also analyzes circadian rhythms of the sleep or activity cycles. This includes the computation of mesor (the mean of the rhythm), the amplitude (peak of the rhythm) and the acrophase (timing of the peak of the rhythm). Those analyses require approximately seven days of data to be most accurate. In those cases, light measurements are also very helpful in many situations [1].

Applications

Regarding our topic, actigraphs can be used not only in PLM patients but also in RLS. There should be software that analyzes the complete circadian disorder, since RLS patients have a tendency toward late sleep onset.

The diagnosis and monitoring of the results, wherever intervention protocol is applied, is an interesting way to have objective data showing the performance of the intervention in the patient´s disorder. They are chronic disorders that can vary from night to night, and actigraphs must be used for at least 7 nights.

In this situation, it is critical that the patient does have a sleep diary in which he/she notes down events during the night, other than situations such as a shower, that the patient eventually takes the actigraphs off. Actigraphs are particular useful for children who do not submit to a full night's polysomnography with electroencephalogram.

It is useful to note that the reliability of estimated sleep time varies considerably depending on the device used, the setting and the specific population being studied. In cases presenting very disturbed sleep, the total sleep time detected by actigraphs correlates to EEG, but not necessarily to minute-by-minute evaluation. There might be other devices with other algorithms, which should ideally prove their reliability; but in general they are quite reliable.

When data are collected in 1-minute epochs and for more than 1 week, it is prudent to download data every week to minimize data loss. Do check the batteries whenever initializing the actigraphs and again during downloading. Battery levels below 90% should be changed because they are likely to fail.

When the devices record light, it is important that the light sensor is not covered by the patient´s clothes. Some devices also have external light sensors that might provide more exact readings.

Editing Actigraphs Data

After downloading the data, the software will provide graphics of activity throughout the hours of the day. Also, the software will provide an estimate of sleep time and all other variables previously discussed. All those data can be edited, based on the patient´s sleep diary. This way, the investigator can manually change intervals for which the device was removed (for instance, when the patient was in the shower) but the patient was awake for certain; otherwise it should be edited as missing data.

References

[1]   Stone KL, Ancoli-Israel S. Actigraphy. In: MH K, T R, WC D, editors. Principles and Practice of Sleep Medicine. Fifth ed. Canada: Elsevier. p. 1668-75.

Chapter 8

Important Updates

Abstract

Science nowadays is updating fast. While preparing and writing this book, researchers were also working on new treatments and papers were published; it is critical for the healthcare professional to stay on top of those updates. The amount of information is overwhelming, and a chapter leading toward some specific sources might help and save time for all health professionals in dealing with RLS and PLM. Also, a number of alternative treatments might be available, so a brief discussion about them will be brought to the reader.

Introduction to Knowledge Sources

The RLS can be found as Willis–Ekbom Disease. A consensus emerged in 2013 from Willis-Ekbom Disease, formerly the Restless Legs Syndrome Foundation and Mayo Clinic [1]. The website is still www.rls.org and it is a useful source of information about the disease. I found the handouts in the treatment option section interesting. The handout of complementary treatments includes a wide range of measures, some of them discussed in this book; some of them are not discussed but can be researched for the future such as osteopathy, cranio sacral therapy, manipulation, and biofeedback, not to mention other kinds of interventions beyond the scope of physiotherapy.

However, the disappointing part of this website is that they only have three accredited centers for RLS treatment in the United States and one center in Austria. If you live in South America or can speak Portuguese, you can consult Consenso Brasileiro Síndrome das Pernas Inquietas, also published in 2013 by the Associação Brasileira de Sono [2]. In this text you can find the authors who study RLS and PLM in Brazil. They discuss the diagnosis, pharmacological and non-pharmacological treatment of RLS/PLM in adults and children, all based on evidence. As mentioned by the main author in his presentation of the consensus during the 2013 Brazilian Sleep Congress, they included only medication allowed in Brazil.

One must be aware that each country might have its own regulatory process to validate medications.

Clinical Set Up: Equipment Needed for Treating RLS and PLM Patients

Apart from learning the treatments, you must also have the equipment to properly care for those RLS and PLM patients. We will consider that the reader might deal with handicapped patients.

- Cycle-ergometer handcycle: if you intend to treat paraplegic patients
- Regular ergometer bike: for idiopathic patients
- Dumbbells
- Treadmill
- Anodyne Therapy or Regular Infrared Light as long as it reaches the parameters used in the research
- Transcutaneous electrical nervous stimulation (TENS)
- Actigraphs: for monitoring the patients

Architecture for the Disabled

Throughout the world, disabled physiotherapy patients will have to overcome more or fewer barriers to arrive at your service: transportation, crossroads, and other situations. Healthcare professionals who intend to deal with handicapped patients must understand their needs and must bear in mind that the patient will not go to a clinic if it is not adapted to their needs.

There are a few basic outlines that you should plan in your clinic that are not so expensive:

1. Accessible ramp for a wheelchair: you can also insert support bars at the side defining it as a pathway. It will prevent other people from putting trash or anything too close to the path for the patient. It must have a small descent angle, being long instead. Because of this small descent angle, you might have to make it with turns instead of a straight line.
2. Handicapped parking: please remember to leave room for the wheelchair.
3. Adapted restroom: these are large spaces, which require a special sink and toilets, with bar support along them of course.
4. Gymnasium: this is a basic structure in physiotherapy clinics: large rooms with no walls are always a standard for physiotherapy clinics. In the gymnasium you can set up the treadmill, the bicycles and the cycle ergometer, besides other material you use for other kinds of patients. You can leave the smaller rooms for infrared application.
5. Evaluation room: this will have to be an isolated larger room. You can have a desk with a computer to download the information from your actigraphs and to evaluate your patients.

Comorbidities and Team Work

Even though other diseases related to RLS are beyond the scope of this book, it is important to remind the reader that RLS patients can also have diabetes, hypertension, myocardial infarction, obesity, stroke, cancer, renal disease, anemia, depression, thyroid disease, and migraine. Those conditions have recently been analyzed and can increase the suffering of RLS patients [3]. It might also be important to those patients to have a proper clinical follow-up.

Education and Awareness

In your country, is RLS and PLM or PLM disorder known by the healthcare professional? In my experience, in Physiotherapy Congress in both Brazil, United States and Canada, physiotherapists have never heard of those disorders. And what about the patients? It seems in the United States people know about the symptoms and have access to medical treatment. Even there, it might take years before RLS is diagnosed. So, the reader of this book must share this knowledge with colleagues and must educate the general population to understand the syndrome.

Manual Therapy as a Super Stretching

I think this article is worth discussing. The authors used a manual therapy technique called straight leg raise with traction to treat RLS. Thirteen subjects (11 female) between the ages of 32–64 completed the study. Subjects completed two questionnaires to quantify the severity of their RLS before treatment was initiated and at the final session. These measures included: the Restless Legs Syndrome Rating Scale (RLSRS) 0–40, an RLS Ordinal Scale, and a Global Rating of Change (GROC) assessments (−7, 0, +7). Patients were treated with RLS bilaterally for a total of four visits on days 1, 3, 8, and 15. Results indicated an RLSRS pre-treatment average of 24.8 (severe) and post-treatment average of 9.2 (mild), representing a 63% improvement from baseline ($p < 0.05$). Ten of 13 subjects reported a GROC of +4 or higher at the final session, indicating at least a moderate improvement in patient status from baseline. Results indicate that following a series of RLS treatments, symptoms were reduced in individuals with idiopathic RLS. A prospective, randomized controlled trial is necessary to evaluate the potential for effectively managing idiopathic RLS symptoms [4]. A probable mechanism of action would be the super strength that this maneuver provides, leading to an amazing increase in the hip flexion range of motion, stretching all the paravertebral musculature and having a neuromuscular response in the spinal cord. The range of improvement in RLS patients is quite amazing. More studies should follow to confirm those findings.

Special Notes for Physiotherapists: Other Sensory and Motor Symptoms in RLS and PLM

This section will provide important insights for physiotherapists dealing with RLS patients. Clinical presentation can involve pain, being a common feature [5]. A discussion about sensory systems and RLS is shown in a comprehensive book about RLS. I insert cramps as a motor feature that might also go hand in hand with PLM. It is important for the physiotherapist to also direct and treat those features accordingly, using regular physiotherapy daily resources. We can consider that cramp is a motor manifestation followed immediately by pain.

The pain epidemiology rates range from 47% to 79% of RLS patients reporting pain. The importance of pain for the quality of life of those patients equates to sleep deprivation and presents the healthcare community with a huge problem to be dealt with. The importance of quality of life for those patients was shown in the REST study (RLS epidemiology, symptom, and treatment survey), in which 16 202 people were evaluated in SF-36, a validated international quality of life instrument. 7% had RLS.

The RLS group presented a strong correlation between the severity of RLS and the physical and mental health-related quality of life in patients (HrQol). In this instrument, two main issues were identified: pain and discomfort in 88% of the patients and 76% presenting sleep disorders.

Other studies used HrQol in RLS to compare to diabetes and depression, showing a similar impairment to depression and diabetes [5, 6]. This has led to a movement toward considering RLS a handicap, which is beyond the scope of this book. The important point for physiotherapists is to evaluate and treat the pain symptoms in those patients. They also have considerable depressive symptoms that can prove an obstacle to willingness to exercise.

Challenges for the Future

We can consider some topics as challenges for the future regarding RLS, PLM and physiotherapy.

- Study new physical treatments already published
- Teach and train other colleagues and patients
- Teach sleep hygiene
- Study the neurological link responsible for their occurrence in SCI
- Study this occurrence in amputees
- Study and deal with this occurrence in fibromyalgia patients

References

[1] Silber MH, Becker PM, Earley C, Garcia-Borreguero D, Ondo WG, editors. Willis-Ekbom Disease Foundation revised consensus statement on the management of restless legs syndrome. *Mayo Clinic Proceedings*; 2013: Elsevier.

[2] RIZZO G. Síndrome das Pernas Inquietas.

[3] Szentkiralyi A, Volzke H, Hoffmann W, Trenkwalder C, Berger K. Multimorbidity and the risk of restless legs syndrome in 2 prospective cohort studies. *Neurology.* 2014.

[4] Dinkins EM, Stevens-Lapsley J. Management of symptoms of Restless Legs Syndrome with use of a traction straight leg raise: A preliminary case series. *Manual therapy.* 2013;18(4):299-302.

[5] Winkelman JW, Gagnon A, Clair AG. Sensory symptoms in restless legs syndrome: the enigma of pain. *Sleep medicine.* 2013;14(10):934-42.

[6] Chaudhuri K, Muzerengi S. Symptoms and health-related quality of life. In: Chaudhuri R, Strambi L-F, Rye D, editors. *Restless Legs Syndrome.* 1. 1 ed. New York: Oxford; 2008. p. 27-34.

Index

E

F

G

U

T

V

W

Y